CAMBRIDGE LIBRARY COLLECTION

Books of enduring scholarly value

History of Medicine

It is sobering to realise that as recently as the year in which On the Origin of Species was published, learned opinion was that diseases such as typhus and cholera were spread by a 'miasma', and suggestions that doctors should wash their hands before examining patients were greeted with mockery by the profession. The Cambridge Library Collection reissues milestone publications in the history of Western medicine as well as studies of other medical traditions. Its coverage ranges from Galen on anatomical procedures to Florence Nightingale's common-sense advice to nurses, and includes early research into genetics and mental health, colonial reports on tropical diseases, documents on public health and military medicine, and publications on spa culture and medicinal plants.

Medical Ethics

A physician and medical reformer enthused by the scientific and cultural progress of the Enlightenment as it took hold in Britain, Thomas Percival (1740–1804) wrote on many topics, but he was particularly concerned about public health issues arising from the factory conditions of the Industrial Revolution. Calling for improved standards of care, he believed that the working poor should be treated the same as wealthy private clients. Following a disastrous dispute in 1792 which closed the Manchester Infirmary's Fever Hospital during an epidemic, Percival was asked to draft regulations on professional medical conduct. In 1794 he privately circulated a tract, *Medical Jurisprudence*, which he later revised for this 1803 publication. Based on Hippocratic and Christian principles, Percival's work is considered the first modern formulation of doctor–patient etiquette. His *Essays Medical and Experimental* (revised edition, 1772–3) and the four volumes of his collected works (1807) are also reissued in this series.

Cambridge University Press has long been a pioneer in the reissuing of out-of-print titles from its own backlist, producing digital reprints of books that are still sought after by scholars and students but could not be reprinted economically using traditional technology. The Cambridge Library Collection extends this activity to a wider range of books which are still of importance to researchers and professionals, either for the source material they contain, or as landmarks in the history of their academic discipline.

Drawing from the world-renowned collections in the Cambridge University Library and other partner libraries, and guided by the advice of experts in each subject area, Cambridge University Press is using state-of-the-art scanning machines in its own Printing House to capture the content of each book selected for inclusion. The files are processed to give a consistently clear, crisp image, and the books finished to the high quality standard for which the Press is recognised around the world. The latest print-on-demand technology ensures that the books will remain available indefinitely, and that orders for single or multiple copies can quickly be supplied.

The Cambridge Library Collection brings back to life books of enduring scholarly value (including out-of-copyright works originally issued by other publishers) across a wide range of disciplines in the humanities and social sciences and in science and technology.

Medical Ethics

Or, a Code of Institutes and Precepts, Adapted to the Professional Conduct of Physicians and Surgeons

Thomas Percival

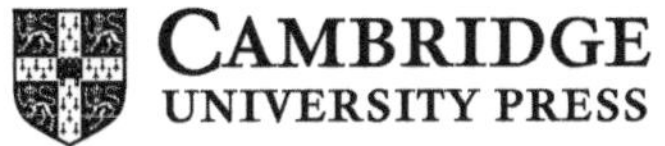

CAMBRIDGE
UNIVERSITY PRESS

University Printing House, Cambridge, CB2 8BS, United Kingdom

Cambridge University Press is part of the University of Cambridge.
It furthers the University's mission by disseminating knowledge in the pursuit of education, learning and research at the highest international levels of excellence.

www.cambridge.org
Information on this title: www.cambridge.org/9781108067225

This edition first published 1803
This digitally printed version 2014

ISBN 978-1-108-06722-5 Paperback

MEDICAL ETHICS;

OR, A CODE OF

Institutes and Precepts,

ADAPTED TO THE

PROFESSIONAL CONDUCT

OF

PHYSICIANS AND SURGEONS;

I. In Hospital Practice.
II. In private, or general Practice.
III. In relation to Apothecaries.
IV. In Cases which may require a knowledge of Law.

To which is added

An Appendix;

containing

A DISCOURSE ON HOSPITAL DUTIES;

ALSO

NOTES AND ILLUSTRATIONS.

BY

THOMAS PERCIVAL, M.D.

F. R. S. AND A. S. LOND. F. R. S. AND R. M. S. EDINB. &c. &c.

Manchester:

PRINTED BY S. RUSSELL,

FOR J. JOHNSON, ST. PAUL'S CHURCH YARD, AND
R. BICKERSTAFF, STRAND, LONDON.

1803.

TO

SIR GEORGE BAKER, BART.

PHYSICIAN TO THEIR MAJESTIES;

FELLOW OF THE ROYAL SOCIETY;

AND

LATE PRESIDENT OF THE COLLEGE OF PHYSICIANS;

&c. &c.

THIS CODE OF

PROFESSIONAL ETHICS;

WHICH HE HAS

HONOURED WITH HIS SANCTION,

AND IMPROVED BY HIS COMMUNICATIONS,

IS GRATEFULLY AND RESPECTFULLY

INSCRIBED,

BY HIS

OBLIGED AND AFFECTIONATE FRIEND,

THE AUTHOR.

TO

E. C. PERCIVAL.

PERMIT me, my dear son, to offer to your acceptance this little Manual of MEDICAL ETHICS. In the composition of it, my thoughts were directed towards your late excellent Brother, with the tenderest impulse of paternal love: And not a single moral rule was framed without a secret view to his designation; and an anxious wish that it might influence his future conduct.

To you, who possess, in no inferior degree, my esteem and attachment; who are prosecuting the

the same studies, and with the same object; my solicitudes are naturally transferred. And I am persuaded, these united considerations will powerfully and permanently operate upon your ingenuous mind.

It is the characteristic of a wise man to act on determinate principles; and of a good man to be assured that they are conformable to rectitude and virtue. The relations in which a physician stands to his patients, to his brethren, and to the public, are complicated, and multifarious; involving much knowledge of human nature, and extensive moral duties. The study of professional Ethics, therefore, cannot fail to invigorate and enlarge your understanding; whilst

the

the observance of the duties which they enjoin, will soften your manners, expand your affections, and form you to that propriety and dignity of conduct, which are essential to the character of a GENTLEMAN. The academical advantages you have enjoyed at Cambridge, and those you now possess in Edinburgh, will qualify you, I trust, for an ample and honourable sphere of action. And I devoutly pray, that the blessing of God may attend all your pursuits; rendering them at once subservient to your own felicity, and the good of your fellow-creatures.

Sensible that I begin to experience the pressure of advancing years, I regard the present publication

cation as the conclusion, in this way, of my professional labours. I may, therefore, without impropriety, claim the privilege of consecrating them to you, as a paternal legacy. And I feel cordial satisfaction in the occasion, of thus testifying the esteem and tenderness with which, whilst life subsists, I shall remain,

Your affectionate friend,

THOMAS PERCIVAL.

Manchester, February 20, 1803.

CONTENTS.

N. B. The Roman Numerals refer to the Sections, and the Figures to the Pages.

PREFACE.—Origin of the work.—Suspension of it.—Farther progress of it.—Addition of supplementary notes and illustrations............................ ..... 1—7.

CHAP. I. *Of professional conduct relative to hospital or other medical charities.*

Duties of hospital physicians and surgeons.—Tenderness.—Steadiness.—Condescension.—Authority. I.—Choice of their attendant physician or surgeon, how far allowable to hospital patients. II.—Feelings and emotions of patients, under critical circumstances, to be duly regarded. III.—No discussion concerning the nature of their case to be entered into before them. IV.—Delicacy in many cases particularly required; and secrecy sometimes to be strictly observed. V.—Moral and religious influence of sickness to be cherished and promoted. VI.—Propriety of suggesting to patients, under certain circumstances, the importance of making their last will and testament. VII.—Parsimony in prescribing wine and drugs of high price reprobated. VIII.—Hospital affairs and occurrences not to be incautiously revealed. IX.—Professional charges to be made only before a meeting of the faculty. X.—Proper discrimination between the medical and chirurgical cases to be strictly adhered to. XI.—What circumstances authorize new remedies and new methods of chirurgical treatment. XII.—Unreserved intercourse should

should subsist between the gentlemen of the faculty; and an account of every case or operation which is rare, curious, or instructive, should be regularly drawn up and preserved. XIII.—Scheme for hospital registers. XIV.—Advantages arising from the scheme. XV.—Close and crowded wards reprobated. XVI.—Establishment of a committee of the gentlemen of the faculty considered. XVII.—Importance of frequent consultations, and the mutual assistance of the physicians and surgeons. XVIII.—Rules to be observed in consultations. XIX.—Rules to be observed respecting operations. XX.—Hospital consultations ought not to be held on Sundays, except in cases of urgent necessity. XXI.—Stated days for operations, often inconvenient and improper. XXII.—Dispensaries. XXIII.—Asylums for female patients labouring under syphilis.—Rules to be observed in lock-hospitals.—XXIV.—Asylums for insanity. XXV.—Modes of acquiring knowledge in the treatment of insanity recommended. XXVI.—Treatment of lunatics—tenderness—indulgence. XXVII.—Boldness of practice sometimes required in cases of mania.—Hospitals for small-pox—Inoculation, &c. &c., require no professional duties not already enumerated. XXVIII.

CHAP. II. *Of professional conduct in private, or general practice.*

Moral rules of conduct, the same with those to be observed towards hospital-patients. I.—The strictest temperance required. II.—Proper conduct to be observed respecting prognostications, and the disclosure of circumstances, to the friends of the patients. III.—Proper conduct respecting interference in cases under the charge of another. IV.—Conduct to be observed towards a physician formerly employed by the patient, but

but not now cousulted. V.—Distinction between the provinces of physic and surgery to be steadily maintained. VI.—Consultations to be promoted in difficult or protracted cases. VII.—Special consultation.—Conduct of the physician called in. VIII.—Theoretical discussions to be avoided in consultations. IX.—Rules for consultations the same with those prescribed to the faculty attending hospitals.—Seniority, how determined. X.—Education of medical men—what influence it ought to have in the consideration of their brethren. XI.—Punctuality in visits of consultation—further rules to be observed. XII.—Visits to the sick not to be unseasonably repeated. XIII.—Rules to be observed with regard to fees, when a physician officiates in the absence, or at the request, of another. XIV.—Importance of adopting some general rule respecting pecuniary acknowledgments. XV.—Medical men and their families, when to be attended gratuitously.—XVI. Peculiar delicacy and attention often required in attendance upon them. XVII.—Attendance on clergymen in narrow circumstances. XVIII.—Consultation by letter. XIX.—Rules to be observed in furnishing certificates. XX.—Use of quack medicines discouraged. XXI.—The dispensing of nostrums reprobated. XXII.—Duty incumbent on individuals to promote the general reputation of the faculty collectively. XXIII.—Rule to be observed in professional controversy and contention. XXIV.—Giving advice gratis. XXV.—Rule to be observed in visiting the patient of another physician. XXVI.—Another case of the same. XXVII.—Review of the treatment and progress of interesting cases recommended. XXVIII.—Moral and religious advice to patients. XXIX.—Observance of the Sabbath, by medical gentlemen, considered. XXX.—Co-operation of young and

and aged practitioners. XXXI.—Period of senescense in physicians considered. XXXII.

CHAP. III. *Of the conduct of physicians to apothecaries.*

Connection between the apothecary and physician. I.—Apothecary often precursor to the physician, and commonly acquainted with the diseases of the family. II.—Rule to be observed in the intercourse and co-operation of the physician and apothecary. III.—Duty and responsibility of the physician. IV.—Particular directions to be observed in visiting country patients with the apothecary. V.—Profits of apothecaries. VI.—Physicians visiting the patients of apothecaries, in their absence, not approved of. VII.—Duty of apothecaries in recommending physicians to families. VIII.—Establishment of funds for the benefit of the widows and children of apothecaries. IX.

CHAP. IV. *Of professional duties in certain cases which require a knowledge of law.*

Medical gentlemen exempt from serving on inquests, juries, &c.; but frequently called upon to exercise duties which require juridical knowledge. I.—Duty of physicians in cases of last will and testament—knowledge of law required. II.—Commissions of lunacy—appointment of a curator. III.—Treatment of lunatics as authorized by law. IV.—Asylums for lunatics subject to strict regulations of law. V.—Opinions given in cases of sudden death. VI.—Justifiable homicide. VII.—Excusable homicide. VIII.—Suicide. IX.—Manslaughter—Murder. X.—Murder of bastard children. XI.—Duelling. XII.—Duty of surgeons with respect to attending a duellist to the field of combat. XIII.—Private and personal duty of physicians with respect to duel—true honour considered. XIV.—Homicide by poison—cases adduced. XV.—Law in cases of rape. XVI.

XVI.—Nuisances defined and considered. XVII.—Duty of medical gentlemen when summoned to attend coroners, migistrates and judges. XVIII.—Importance to gentlemen of the faculty of settling their opinions concerning the right of magistrates to inflict capital punishment —The limits prescribed to the exercise of the right; and the duty of giving full efficiency to law. XIX.—Cautions relative to professional testimony in cases of peculiar malignity. XX.

A Discourse on Hospital Duties.

Addresses.—I. To the faculty, p. 120.—II. To the officers and superintendants, p. 126.—III. To the clergy, p. 130.—IV. To the trustees of the Infirmary at Liverpool, p. 132.

Notes and Illustrations.

Note.	Page.
I. Hospital at Manchester	135
II. Distribution of printed copies of the Medical Ethics	139
III. Situation, construction and government of hospitals	140
IV. House of reception for patients ill of contagious fevers	147
V. Caution or temerity in practice	152
VI. Temperance of physicians	154
VII. A physician should be the minister of hope and comfort to the sick.—Enquiry, how far it is justifiable to violate truth for the supposed benefit of the patient	156
VIII. The practice of prior physicians should be treated with candour, and justified so far as truth and probity will permit	168
IX. Theoretical discussions should be generally avoided	169

X. Regular

X. Regular academical education....................... 170
XI. Pecuniary acknowledgments....................... 174
XII. Public worship; scepticism and infidelity...... 179
XIII. Union and consultation of senior and junior physicians.. 200
XIV. Retirement from practice—when—Letters from Dr. Heberden; and Sir G. Baker, Bart.. 201
XV. Partial insanity with general intelligence—Lucid interval.. 206
XVI. Duelling.—Letter from Dr. Franklin.......... 214
XVII. Punishment of the crime of rape.—Disney's views of ancient laws against immorality, &c.—Eden's principles of penal law............. 228
XVIII. Uncertainty in the external signs of rape—Communication from Mr. Ward................. 231
XIX. The smoke from large works a nuisance—Coalbrook-Dale...................................... 234
XX. Discourse on Hospital Duties; by the Rev. T. B. Percival, LL. B.—Brief memoirs of him 238
XXI. The salutary connections of sickness not to be rashly dissolved—Cautions concerning the removal of patients into an hospital—Extracts from the Memoirs of the Rev. Newcome Cappe 239
XXII. Duty of hospital trustees in electing the medical officers of the charity—Advertisement of the governors of the Salisbury Infirmary.—Memorial to the trustees of the Manchester Infirmary.. 243

ERRATA.

Reference to Note VII. wanting - - - - - Page 32
For *guilt* manslaughter—read *of*—line 10 - - - - - 78
For Note XVII—read Note XVI. - - - - - - - 93
For Note XVI—read Note XVII. - - - - - - - 99
For Note XVII—read Note XVIII. - - - - - - 103
For *or*—read *for*—line 26 - - - - - - - - - - 163
For *decripitude*—read *decrepitude*—line 4 - - - - 197

PREFACE.

THE first chapter of the following work was composed in the spring of 1792, at the request of the physicians and surgeons of the Manchester Infirmary: And the substance of it constitutes the code of laws, by which the practice of that comprehensive institution is now governed. (*a*) The author was afterwards induced, by an earnest desire to promote the honour and advancement of his profession, to enlarge the plan of his undertaking, and to frame a general system of MEDICAL ETHICS; that the official conduct, and mutual intercourse of the faculty, might be regulated by precise and acknowledged principles of urbanity and rectitude. Printed copies of the scheme were, therefore, distributed amongst his numerous correspondents;

(*a*) See Notes and Illustrations, No. I.

dents; by most of whom it was warmly encouraged; and by many of them was honoured with valuable suggestions for its improvement. (*b*)

Whilst the author was thus extending his views, and carrying on his work with ardour, he lost the strongest incentive to its prosecution, by the death of a beloved son, who had nearly completed the course of his academical education; and whose talents, acquirements, and virtues, promised to render him an ornament to the healing art. This melancholy event was followed, not many years afterwards, by a second family loss equally afflictive; and the design has ever since been wholly suspended. The author now resumes it, animated by the hope that it may prove beneficial to another son, who has lately exchanged the pursuits of general science at Cambridge, for the study of medicine at Edinburgh: He feels at the same time, impressed with the conviction, that the languor

(*b*) See Notes and Illuftrations, No. II.

languor of sorrow becomes culpable, when it obstructs the offices of an active vocation. "I hold every man," says Lord Bacon, in the preface to his Elements of the Common Laws of England, "a debtor to his profes-"sion; from the which as men of course "do seek to receive countenance and "profit, so ought they of duty to en-"deavour themselves, by way of amends, "to be a help and ornament thereunto. "This is performed, in some degree, by the "honest and liberal practice of a pro-"fession; when men shall carry a respect "not to descend into any course that is "corrupt and unworthy thereof; and pre-"serve themselves free from the abuses "wherewith the same profession is noted "to be infected: But much more is this "performed, if a man be able to visit and "strengthen the roots and foundation of the "science itself; thereby not only gracing "it in reputation and dignity, but also "amplifying it in profession and substance."

 It

It was the author's original intention to have treated of the POWERS, PRIVILEGES, HONOURS, and EMOLUMENTS of the FACULTY. But he now conceives, that this would lead him into a field of investigation too wide and digressive; and therefore chooses to confine himself to what more strictly belongs to Medical Ethics.

To these institutes he has annexed an Anniversary Discourse, delivered by the late Rev. Thomas Bassnett Percival, LL. B. before the president, and governors of the Infirmary, at Liverpool. As it is an address to the gentlemen of the faculty, the officers, the clergy, and the trustees of the charity, on their respective hospital duties, by one competent to the subject from his early studies, it cannot but be deemed sufficiently appropriate to the present work, exclusively of a father's claim to the privilege of its insertion.

The aphoristic form of this code of Medical Ethics, though adapted to such an undertaking, forbids in a great measure, all digression

gression; and even precludes the discussion of many interesting points, nearly connected with the subject. SUPPLEMENTARY NOTES AND ILLUSTRATIONS, therefore, are necessary to the completion of the author's plan: And he trusts the candid reader will grant him the liberty of thus stating his opinions more at large; of rectifying misconceptions, to which the brevity essential to the work may give rise; and of correcting whatever subsequent reflection, or the judicious observations of his friends, may discover to be erroneous.

A considerable portion of these sheets was communicated to the REV. THOMAS GISBORNE, M. A. whilst engaged in the composition of his ENQUIRY into the DUTIES of MEN; a work that reflects the highest honour on the abilities, and philanthropy of the author; and which may be justly regarded as the most complete system, extant, of PRACTICAL ETHICS. The chapter concerning physicians contains a reference to these institutes, expressed

pressed in the most gratifying terms of friendship: And it treats so largely of the duties of the faculty, as to seem, at first view, to supersede the use of the present manual. But the two publications differ not only in their plan, but in many of their leading objects; and it may be hoped they will rather illustrate than interfere with each other. The same remarks may be applied to the excellent lectures of Dr. Gregory. Even the STATUTA MORALIA of the college of physicians, whatever merit or authority they possess, are not sufficiently comprehensive for the existing sphere of medical and chirurgical duty: And by the few regulations which they establish, they tacitly sanction the recommendation of a fuller and more adequate code of professional offices.

Copies of the former unfinished impression of this work have been transmitted to the libraries of several Infirmaries, in different parts of the kingdom: And the author has reason to hope, that they have contributed to excite attention

attention to the subject of hospital police. Amongst other pleasing proofs of this truth, he refers with peculiar satisfaction to the late publications of his friends, Sir G. O. Paul, Bart. and Dr. Clark, of Newcastle-upon-Tyne.

This work was originally entitled "MEDICAL JURISPRUDENCE"; but some friends having objected to the term JURISPRUDENCE, it has been changed to ETHICS. According to the definition of Justinian, however, Jurisprudence may be understood to include moral injunctions as well as positive ordinances. *Juris præcepta sunt hæc; honestè vivere; alterum non lædere; suum cuique tribuere.* INST. JUSTIN: LIB. I. p. 3.

MANCHESTER, FEB. 15, 1803.

— QUICQUID DIGNUM SAPIENTE BONO-QUE EST.

HOR. Lib. I. Ep. IV.

MEDICAL ETHICS;

OR

A CODE OF INSTITUTES AND PRECEPTS,

ADAPTED TO THE

PROFESSIONAL CONDUCT

OF

PHYSICIANS AND SURGEONS.

CHAPTER I.

OF PROFESSIONAL CONDUCT, RELATIVE TO HOSPITALS, OR OTHER MEDICAL CHARITIES.

I. HOSPITAL PHYSICIANS and SURGEONS should minister to the sick, with due impressions of the importance of their office; reflecting that the ease, the health, and the lives of those committed to their charge depend on their skill, attention, and fidelity. They should study, also, in their deportment, so to unite *tenderness* with *steadiness*, and *condescension* with *authority*, as to inspire the minds of their patients with gratitude, respect, and confidence.

 II. The

II. The *choice* of a *physician* or *surgeon* cannot be allowed to hospital patients, consistently with the regular and established succession of medical attendance. Yet personal confidence is not less important to the comfort and relief of the sick-poor, than of the rich under similar circumstances: And it would be equally just and humane, to enquire into and to indulge their partialities, by occasionally calling into consultation the favourite practitioner. The rectitude and wisdom of this conduct will be still more apparent, when it is recollected that patients in hospitals not unfrequently request their discharge, on a deceitful plea of having received relief; and afterwards procure another recommendation, that they may be admitted under the physician or surgeon of their choice. Such practices involve in them a degree of falshood; produce unnecessary trouble; and may be the occasion of irreparable loss of time in the treatment of diseases.

III. The *feelings* and *emotions* of the patients, under critical circumstances, require to be known and to be attended to, no less than the symptoms of their diseases. Thus, extreme *timidity*, with respect to venæsection, contraindicates its use, in certain cases and constitutions. Even the *prejudices* of the sick are not to be contemned, or opposed with harshness. For though silenced by authority, they will operate secretly and forcibly on the mind, creating fear, anxiety, and watchfulness.

IV. As misapprehension may magnify real evils, or create imaginary ones, no *discussion* concerning the nature of the case should be entered into before the patients, either with the house surgeon, the pupils of the hospitals, or any medical visitor.

V. In the large wards of an Infirmary the patients should be interrogated concerning their complaints, in a *tone* of *voice* which cannot be *overheard*. *Secrecy*, also, when required by peculiar circumstances, should be strictly observed. And females should always be treated with the most scrupulous *delicacy*. To neglect or to sport with their feelings is cruelty; and every wound thus inflicted tends to produce a callousness of mind, a contempt of decorum, and an insensibility to modesty and virtue. Let these considerations be forcibly and repeatedly urged on the hospital pupils.

VI. The *moral* and *religious influence* of sickness is so favourable to the best interests of men and of society, that it is justly regarded as an important object in the establishment of every hospital. The *institutions* for promoting it should, therefore, be encouraged by the physicians and surgeons, whenever seasonable opportunities occur. And by pointing out these to the officiating clergyman, the sacred offices will be performed with propriety, discrimination, and greater certainty of success. The character of a physician is usually remote either from superstition or enthusiasm: And the aid, which he is now exhorted to give, will tend to their exclusion from the sick wards of the hospital, where their effects have often been known to be not only baneful, but even fatal.

VII. It is one of the circumstances which softens the lot of the poor, that they are exempt from the solicitudes attendant on the disposal of property. Yet there are exceptions to this observation; And it may be necessary that an hospital patient, on the bed of sickness and death, should be reminded, by some friendly monitor, of the importance of a *last will* and *testament* to his wife, children, or relatives, who, otherwise, might be deprived of his effects, of his expected prize money, or of some future residuary legacy. This kind office

office will be best performed by the house-surgeon, whose frequent attendance on the sick diminishes their reserve, and entitles him to their familiar confidence. And he will doubtless regard the performance of it as a duty. For whatever is right to be done, and cannot by another be so well done, has the full force of moral and personal obligation.

VIII. The physicians and surgeons should not suffer themselves to be restrained, by parsimonious considerations, from prescribing *wine*, and *drugs* even of *high price*, when required in diseases of extraordinary malignity and danger. The efficacy of every medicine is proportionate to its purity and goodness; and on the degree of these properties, *cæteris paribus*, both the cure of the sick, and the speediness of its accomplishment must depend. But when drugs of inferior quality are employed, it is requisite to administer them in larger doses, and to continue the use of them a longer period of time; circumstances which, probably, more than counterbalance any savings in their original price. If the case, however, were far otherwise, no œconomy, of a fatal tendency, ought to be admitted into institutions, founded on principles of the purest beneficence, and which, in this age and country, when

when well conducted, can never want contributions adequate to their liberal support.

IX. The medical gentlemen of every charitable institution are, in some degree, responsible for, and the guardians of, the honour of each other. No physician or surgeon, therefore, should *reveal* occurrences in the hospital, which may injure the reputation of any one of his colleagues; except under the restriction contained in the succeeding article.

X. No *professional charge* should be made by a physician or surgeon, either publicly or privately, against any associate, without previously laying the complaint before the gentlemen of the faculty belonging to the institution, that they may judge concerning the reasonableness of its grounds, and the measures to be adopted.

XI. A proper *discrimination* being established in all hospitals between the *medical* and *chirurgical cases*, it should be faithfully adhered to, by the physicians and surgeons, on the admission of patients.

XII. Whenever cases occur, attended with circumstances not heretofore observed, or in which the ordinary modes of practice have been attempted without success, it is for the public good, and in an especial degree advantageous

vantageous to the poor (who, being the most numerous class of society, are the greatest beneficiaries of the healing art) that *new remedies* and *new methods* of *chirurgical treatment* should be devised. But in the accomplishment of this salutary purpose, the gentlemen of the faculty should be scrupulously and conscientiously governed by sound reason, just analogy, or well authenticated facts. And no such trials should be instituted, without a previous consultation of the physicians or surgeons, according to the nature of the case.

XIII. To advance professional improvement, a friendly and unreserved *intercourse* should subsist between the gentlemen of the faculty, with a free communication of whatever is extraordinary or interesting in the course of their hospital practice. And an *account* of every *case* or *operation*, which is rare, curious, or instructive, should be drawn up by the physician or surgeon, to whose charge it devolves, and entered in a register kept for the purpose, but open only to the physicians and surgeons of the charity.

XIV. *Hospital registers* usually contain only a simple report of the number of patients admitted and discharged. By adopting a more comprehensive plan, they might be rendered subservient

subservient to medical science, and beneficial to mankind. The following sketch is offered, with deference, to the gentlemen of the faculty. Let the register consist of three tables; the first specifying the number of patients admitted, cured, relieved, discharged, or dead; the second the several diseases of the patients, with their events; the third the sexes, ages, and occupations of the patients. The ages should be reduced into classes; and the tables adapted to the four divisions of the year. By such an institution, the increase or decrease of sickness; the attack, progress, and cessation of epidemics; the comparative healthiness of different situations, climates, and seasons; the influence of particular trades and manufactures on health and life; with many other curious circumstances, not more interesting to physicians than to the community, would be ascertained with sufficient precision.

XV. By the adoption of the *register*, recommended in the foregoing article, physicians and surgeons would obtain a clearer insight into the comparative success of their hospital and private practice; and would be incited to a diligent investigation of the causes of such difference. In particular diseases it will be found to subsist in a very remarkable

degree:

degree: And the discretionary power of the physician or surgeon, in the admission of patients, could not be exerted with more justice or humanity, than in refusing to consign to lingering suffering, and almost certain death, a numerous class of patients, inadvertently recommended as objects of these charitable institutions. "In "judging of diseases with regard to the pro-"priety of their reception into hospitals," says an excellent writer, "the following general "circumstances are to be considered:"

"Whether they be capable of speedy relief; "because, as it is the intention of charity to "relieve as great a number as possible, a "quick change of objects is to be wished; "and also because the inbred disease of hos-"pitals will almost inevitably creep, in some "degree, upon one who continues a long "time in them, but will rarely attack one, "whose stay is short.

"Whether they require in a particular man-"ner the superintendence of skilful persons, "either on account of their acute and dan-"gerous nature, or any singularity or intri-"cacy attending them, or erroneous opinions "prevailing among the common people con-"cerning their treatment.

"Whether they be contagious, or subject "in a peculiar degree to taint the air, and "generate pestilential diseases.

"Whether a fresh and pure air be peculiarly requisite for their cure, and they "be remarkably injured by any vitiation of "it."*

XVI. But no precautions relative to the reception of patients, who labour under maladies incapable of relief, contagious in their nature, or liable to be aggravated by confinement in an impure atmosphere, can obviate the evils arising from *close wards*, and the false œconomy of crowding a number of persons into the least possible space. There are inbred diseases which it is the duty of the physician or surgeon to prevent, as far as lies in his power, by a strict and persevering attention to the whole medical polity of the hospital. This comprehends the discrimination of cases admissible, air, diet, cleanliness, and drugs; each of which articles should be subjected to a rigid scrutiny, at stated periods of time. *(c)*

XVII. The establishment of a *committee* of the *gentlemen* of the *faculty*, to be held monthly,

* See Dr. Aikin's Thoughts on Hospitals, p. 21.

(*c*) See Notes and Illuſtrations, No. III.

monthly, would tend to facilitate this interesting investigation, and to accomplish the most important objects of it. By the free communication of remarks, various improvements would be suggested; by the regular discussion of them, they would be reduced to a definite and consistent form; and by the authority of united suffrages, they would have full influence over the governors of the charity. The exertions of individuals, however benevolent or judicious, often give rise to jealousy; are opposed by those who have not been consulted; and prove inefficient by wanting the collective energy of numbers.

XVIII. The harmonious intercourse, which has been recommended to the gentlemen of the faculty, will naturally produce *frequent consultations*, viz. of the physicians on medical cases, of the surgeons on chirurgical cases, and of both united in cases of a compound nature, which falling under the department of each, may admit of elucidation by the reciprocal aid of the two professions.

XIX. In consultations on medical cases, the junior physician present should *deliver* his *opinion* first, and the others in the progressive order of their seniority. The same order should be observed in chirurgical cases; and a majority should be decisive in both: But if the numbers be equal, the decision should rest with the physician or surgeon, under whose care the patient is placed. No decision, however, should restrain the acting practitioner from making such variations in the mode of treatment, as future contingences may require, or a farther insight into the nature of the disorder may shew to be expedient.

XX. In consultations on mixed cases, the junior surgeon should *deliver* his *opinion* first, and his brethren afterwards in succession, according to progressive seniority. The junior physician present should deliver his opinion after the senior surgeon; and the other physicians in the order above prescribed.

XXI. In every consultation, the case to be considered should be *concisely stated* by the physician or surgeon, who requests the aid of his brethren. The opinions relative to it should be delivered with brevity, agreeably to the preceding arrangement, and the decisions collected in the same order. The order of seniority, among the physicians and surgeons, may be regulated by the dates of their respective appointments in the hospital.

XXII. Due *notice* should be given of a consultation, and no person admitted to it, except

except the physicians and surgeons of the hospital, and the house-surgeon, without the unanimous consent of the gentlemen present. If an examination of the patient be previously necessary, the particular circumstances of danger or difficulty should be carefully concealed from him, and every just precaution used to guard him from anxiety or alarm.

XXIII. No important *operation* should be determined upon, without a consultation of the physicians and surgeons, and the acquiescence of a majority of them. Twenty-four hours notice should be given of the proposed operation, except in dangerous accidents, or when peculiar circumstances occur, which may render delay hazardous. The presence of a *spectator* should not be allowed during an operation, without the express permission of the operator. All extra-official interference in the management of it should be forbidden. A decorous *silence* ought to be observed. It may be humane and salutary, however, for one of the attending physicians or surgeons to speak occasionally to the patient; to comfort him under his sufferings; and to give him assurance, if consistent with truth, that the operation

operation goes on well, and promises a speedy and successful termination.*

As a Hospital is the best school for practical surgery, it would be liberal and beneficial to invite, in rotation, two surgeons of the town, who do not belong to the institution, to be present at each operation.

XXIV. Hospital consultations ought not to be held on Sundays, except in cases of urgent necessity; and on such occasions an hour should be appointed, which does not interfere with attendance on public worship.

XXV. It is an established usage, in some hospitals, to have a *stated day* in the week for the performance of operations. But this may occasion improper delay, or equally unjustifiable anticipation. When several operations are to take place in succession, one patient should not have his mind agitated by the knowledge of the sufferings of another. The surgeon should change his apron, when besmeared; and the table or instruments should be

* The substance of the five preceding articles (XIX. XX. XXI. XXII. XXIII.) was suggested by Dr. Ferriar and Mr. Simmons, at the time when I was desired, by them and my other colleagues, to frame a code of rules for the Manchester Infirmary. The additions, now made, are intended to adapt them to general use.

be freed from all marks of blood, and every thing that may excite terror.

XXVI. DISPENSARIES afford the widest sphere for the treatment of diseases, comprehending, not only such as ordinarily occur, but those which are so infectious, malignant, and fatal, as to be excluded from admission into Infirmaries. Happily, also, they neither tend to counteract that spirit of independence, which should be sedulously fostered in the poor, nor to preclude the practical exercise of those relative duties, "the charities of father, son, and brother," which constitute the strongest moral bonds of society. Being institutions less splendid and expensive than hospitals, they are well adapted to towns of moderate size; and might even be established, without difficulty, in populous country districts. Physicians and surgeons, in such situations, have generally great influence: And it would be truly honourable to exert it in a cause subservient to the interests of medical science, of commerce, and of philanthropy. *(d)*

The duties which devolve on gentlemen of the faculty, engaged in the conduct of Dispensaries, are so nearly similar to those of hospital physicians and surgeons, as to be comprehended

(d) See Notes and Illustrations, No. IV.

prehended under the same professional and moral rules. But greater *authority* and greater *condescension* will be found requisite in domestic attendance on the poor. And human nature must be intimately studied, to acquire that full ascendancy over the prejudices, the caprices, and the passions of the sick, and of their relatives, which is essential to medical success.

XXVII. Hospitals, appropriated to particular maladies, are established in different places, and claim both the patronage and the aid of the gentlemen of the faculty. To an ASYLUM for FEMALE PATIENTS, labouring under SYPHILIS, it is to be lamented that discouragements have been too often and successfully opposed. Yet whoever reflects on the variety of diseases to which the human body is incident, will find that a considerable part of them are derived from immoderate passions, and vicious indulgencies. Sloth, intemperance, and irregular desires are the great sources of those evils, which contract the duration, and imbitter the enjoyment of life. But humanity, whilst she bewails the vices of mankind, incites us to alleviate the miseries which flow from them. And it may be proved that a LOCK HOSPITAL is an institution founded on the most benevolent

lent principles, consonant to sound policy, and favourable to reformation and to virtue. It provides relief for a painful and loathsome distemper, which contaminates, in its progress, the innocent as well as the guilty, and extends its baneful influence to future generations. It restores to virtue and to religion those votaries whom pleasure has seduced, or villany betrayed; and who now feel, by sad experience, that ruin, misery, and disgrace *are the wages of sin.* Over such objects pity sheds the generous tear; austerity softens into forgiveness; and benevolence expands at the united pleas of frailty, penitence, and wretchedness.*

No *peculiar rules* of conduct are requisite in the medical attendance on LOCK HOSPITALS. But as these institutions must, from the nature of their object, be in a great measure shut from the inspection of the public, it will behove the faculty to consider themselves as responsible, in an extraordinary degree, for their right government; that the moral, no less than the medical purposes of such esta-

 blishments

* See two Reports, intended to promote the establishment of a Lock Hospital in Manchester, in the year 1774, inserted in the author's Essays Medical, Philosophical, and Experimental. Vol. II. p. 263. 4th Edit.

blishments, may be fully answered. The strictest decorum should be observed in the conduct towards the female patients; no young pupils should be admitted into the house; every ministring office should be performed by nurses properly instructed; and books adapted to the moral improvement of the patients should be put into their hands, and given them on their discharge. To provide against the danger of urgent want, a small sum of money, and decent clothes should at this time be dispensed to them; and, when practicable, some mode should be pointed out of obtaining a reputable livelihood.

XXVIII. ASYLUMS for INSANITY possess accommodations and advantages, of which the poor must, in all circumstances, be destitute; and which no private family, however opulent, can provide. Of these schemes of benevolence all classes of men may have equal occasion to participate the benefits; for human nature itself becomes the mournful object of such institutions. Other diseases leave man a rational and moral agent, and sometimes improve both the faculties of the head, and the affections of the heart. But lunacy subverts the whole rational and moral character; extinguishes every tender charity; and excludes the degraded sufferer from all the enjoyments and advantages

tages of social intercourse. Painful is the office of a physician, when he is called upon to minister to such humiliating objects of distress: Yet great must be his felicity, when he can render himself instrumental, under providence, in the restoration of reason, and in the renewal of the lost image of God. Let no one, however, promise himself this divine privilege, if he be not deeply skilled in the philosophy of human nature. For though casual success may sometimes be the result of empirical practice, the *medicina mentis* can only be administered with steady efficacy by him, who, to a knowledge of the animal œconomy, and of the physical causes which regulate or disturb its movements, unites an intimate acquaintance with the laws of association; the controul of fancy over judgment; the force of habit; the direction and comparative strength of opposite passions; and the reciprocal dependences and relations of the moral and intellectual powers of man.

XXIX. Even thus qualified with the prerequisite attainments, the physician will find that he has a new region of medical science to explore. For it is a circumstance to be regretted, both by the faculty and the public, that the various diseases which are classed

 under

under the title of insanity, remain less understood than any others with which mankind are visited. Hospital institutions furnish the best means of acquiring more accurate knowledge of their causes, nature, and cure. But this information cannot be attained, to any satisfactory extent, by the ordinary attention to single and unconnected cases The synthetic plan should be adopted; and a regular *journal* should be kept of every species of the malady which occurs, arranged under proper heads, with a full detail of its rise, progress, and termination; of the remedies administered, and of their effects in its several stages. The age, sex, occupation, mode of life, and if possible hereditary constitution of each patient should be noted: And, when the event proves fatal, the brain, and other organs affected should be carefully examined, and the appearances on dissection minutely inserted in the journal. A register like this, in the course of a few years, would afford the most interesting and authentic documents, the want of which, on a late melancholy occasion, was felt and regretted by the whole kingdom.

XXX. Lunatics are, in a great measure, secluded from the observation of those who

are

are interested in their good treatment; and their complaints of ill-usage are so often false or fanciful, as to obtain little credit or attention, even when well founded. The physician, therefore, must feel himself under the strictest obligation of honour, as well as of humanity, to secure to these unhappy sufferers all the *tenderness* and *indulgence*, compatible with steady and effectual government.

XXXI. Certain cases of *mania* seem to require a *boldness of practice*, which a young physician of sensibility may feel a reluctance to adopt. On such occasions he must not yield to timidity, but fortify his mind by the councils of his more experienced brethren of the faculty. Yet with this aid, it is more consonant to probity to err on the side of caution than of temerity. *(e)*

Hospitals for the small-pox, for inoculation, for cancers, &c. &c. are established in different places; but require no professional duties, which are not included under, or deducible from, the precepts already delivered.

CHAP.

(e) See Notes, and Illustrations, No. V.

CHAPTER II.

OF PROFESSIONAL CONDUCT IN PRIVATE, OR GENERAL PRACTICE.

I. THE *moral rules of conduct*, prescribed towards hospital patients, should be fully adopted in private or general practice. Every case, committed to the charge of a physician or surgeon, should be treated with attention, steadiness, and humanity: Reasonable indulgence should be granted to the mental imbecility and caprices of the sick: Secrecy, and delicacy when required by peculiar circumstances, should be strictly observed. And the familiar and confidential intercourse, to which the faculty are admitted in their professional visits, should be used with discretion, and with the most scrupulous regard to fidelity and honour.

II. The strictest *temperance* should be deemed incumbent on the faculty; as the practice both of physic and surgery at all times requi es the exercise of a clear and vigorous understanding: And on emergencies, for which no professional man should be unprepared,

pared, a steady hand, an acute eye, and an unclouded head, may be essential to the well being, and even to the life, of a fellow-creature. Philip of Macedon reposed with entire security on the vigilance and attention of his General Parmenio. In his hours of mirth and conviviality he was wont to say, "Let us "drink, my friends; we may do it with "safety, for Parmenio never drinks!" The moral of this story is sufficiently obvious when applied to the faculty; but it should certainly be construed with great limitation by their patients. *(f)*

III. A physician should not be forward to make gloomy prognostications; because they savour of empiricism, by magnifying the importance of his services in the treatment or cure of the disease. But he should not fail, on proper occasions, to give to the friends of the patient, timely notice of danger, when it really occurs, and even to the patient himself, if absolutely necessary. This office, however, is so peculiarly alarming, when executed by him, that it ought to be declined, whenever it can be assigned to any other person of sufficient judgment and delicacy. For the physician

(f) See Notes and Illustrations, No. VI.

sician should be the minister of hope and comfort to the sick; that by such cordials to the drooping spirit, he may smooth the bed of death; revive expiring life; and counteract the depressing influence of those maladies, which rob the philosopher of fortitude, and the Christian of consolation.

IV. *Officious interference*, in a case under the charge of another, should be carefully avoided. No meddling inquiries should be made concerning the patient; no unnecessary hints given, relative to the nature or treatment of his disorder; nor any selfish conduct pursued, that may directly or indirectly tend to diminish the trust reposed in the physician or surgeon employed. Yet though the character of a professional busy-body, whether from thoughtlessness or craft, is highly reprehensible, there are occasions which not only justify but require a spirited interposition. When artful ignorance grossly imposes on credulity; when neglect puts to hazard an important life; or rashness threatens it with still more imminent danger; a medical neighbour, friend, or relative, apprized of such facts, will justly regard his interference as a duty. But he ought to be careful that the information, on which he acts, is well founded; that his motives are pure and honourable:

nourable; and that his judgment of the measures pursued is built on experience and practical knowledge, not on speculative or theoretical differences of opinion. The particular circumstances of the case will suggest the most proper mode of conduct. In general, however, a personal and confidential application to the gentlemen of the faculty concerned, should be the first step taken, and afterwards, if necessary, the transaction may be communicated to the patient or to his family.

V. When a physician or surgeon is called to a patient, who has been before under the care of another gentleman of the faculty, a consultation with him should be even proposed, though he may have discontinued his visits: His practice, also, should be treated with candour, and justified, so far as probity and truth will permit. For the want of success in the primary treatment of a case, is no impeachment of professional skill or knowledge; and it often serves to throw light on the nature of a disease, and to suggest to the subsequent practitioner more appropriate means of relief. *(g)*

VI. In large and opulent towns, the *distinction* between the *provinces* of *physic* and *surgery*

(g) See Notes and Illuſtrations, No. VIII.

surgery should be steadily maintained. This distinction is sanctioned both by reason and experience. It is founded on the nature and objects of the two professions; on the education and acquirements requisite for their most beneficial and honourable exercise; and tends to promote the complete cultivation and advancement of each. For the division of skill and labour is no less advantageous in the liberal than in the mechanic arts: And both physic and surgery are so comprehensive, and yet so far from perfection, as separately to give full scope to the industry and genius of their respective professors. Experience has fully evinced the benefits of the discrimination recommended, which is established in every well regulated hospital, and is thus expressly authorized by the faculty themselves, and by those who have the best opportunities of judging of the proper application of the healing art. No physician or surgeon, therefore, should adopt more than one denomination, or assume any rank or privileges different from those of his order.

VII. *Consultations* should be *promoted*, in difficult or protracted cases, as they give rise to confidence, energy, and more enlarged views

in

in practice. On such occasions no rivalship or jealousy should be indulged: Candour, probity, and all due respect should be exercised towards the physician or surgeon first engaged: And as he may be presumed to be best acquainted with the patient and with his family, he should deliver all the medical directions agreed upon, though he may not have precedency in seniority or rank. It should be the province, however, of the senior physician, first to propose the necessary questions to the sick, but without excluding his associate from the privilege of making farther enquiries, to satisfy himself, or to elucidate the case.

VIII. As circumstances sometimes occur to render a *special consultation* desirable, when the continued attendance of another physician or surgeon might be objectionable to the patient, the gentleman of the faculty, whose assistance is required, in such cases, should pay only two or three visits; and sedulously guard against all future unsolicited interference. For this consultation a double gratuity may reasonably be expected from the patient, as it will be found to require an extraordinary portion both of time and attention.

In medical practice, it is not an unfrequent occurrence, that a physician is hastily summoned, through the anxiety of the family, or the solicitation of friends, to visit a patient, who is under the regular direction of another physician, to whom notice of this call has not been given. Under such circumstances, no change in the treatment of the sick person should be made, till a previous consultation with the stated physician has taken place, unless the lateness of the hour precludes meeting, or the symptoms of the case are too pressing to admit of delay.

IX. *Theoretical discussions* should be avoided in consultations, as occasioning perplexity and loss of time. For there may be much diversity of opinion, concerning speculative points, with perfect agreement in those modes of practice, which are founded not on hypothesis, but on experience and observation. *(h)*

X. The rules prescribed for hospital consultations, may be adopted in private or general practice.* And the *seniority* of a physician may be determined by the period of his public and acknowledged practice as a physician, and that of a surgeon by the period of his practice as a surgeon, in the place where each

(h) See Notes and Illustrations, No. IX.

* See articles xix. xx. xxi. Chap. I.

each resides. This arrangement, being clear and obvious, is adapted to remove all grounds of dispute amongst medical gentlemen: And it secures the regular continuance of the order of precedency, established in every town, which might otherwise be liable to troublesome interruptions by new settlers, perhaps not long stationary.

XI. A regular *academical education* furnishes the only presumptive evidence of professional ability, and is so honourable and beneficial, that it gives a just claim to pre-eminence among physicians, in proportion to the degree in which it has been enjoyed and improved: Yet as it is not indispensably necessary to the attainment of knowledge, skill, and experience, they who have really acquired, in a competent measure, such qualifications, without its advantages, should not be fastidiously excluded from the privileges of fellowship. In consultations, especially, as the good of the patient is the sole object in view, and is often dependent on personal confidence, the aid of an intelligent practitioner ought to be received with candour and politeness, and his advice

advice adopted, if agreeable to sound judgment and truth. *(i)*

XII. *Punctuality* should be observed in the visits of the faculty, when they are to hold consultation together. But as this may not always be practicable, the physician or surgeon, who first arrives at the place of appointment, should wait five minutes for his associate, before his introduction to the patient, that the unnecessary repetition of questions may be avoided: No visits should be made but in concert, or by mutual agreement: No statement or discussion of the case should take place before the patient or his friends, except in the presence of each of the attending gentlemen of the faculty, and by common consent: And no *prognostications* should be delivered, which are not the result of previous deliberation and concurrence.

XIII. *Visits* to the sick should not be *unseasonably repeated;* because, when too frequent, they tend to diminish the authority of the physician, to produce instability in his practice, and to give rise to such occasional indulgences, as are subversive of all medical regimen.

Sir William Temple has asserted, that "an "honest physician is excused for leaving his "patient,

(i) See Notes and Illustrations, No. X.

" patient, when he finds the disease growing " desperate, and can, by his attendance, ex- " pect only to receive his fees, without any " hopes or appearance of deserving them." But this allegation is not well founded: For the offices of a physician may continue to be highly useful to the patient, and comforting to the relatives around him, even in the last period of a fatal malady; by obviating despair, by alleviating pain, and by soothing mental anguish. To decline attendance, under such circumstances, would be sacrificing, to fanciful delicacy and mistaken liberality, that moral duty which is independent of, and far superior to, all pecuniary appreciation.

XIV. Whenever a physician or surgeon *officiates* for another, who is sick or absent, during any considerable length of time, he should receive the fees accruing from such additional practice: But if this fraternal act be of short duration, it should be gratuitously performed; with an observance always of the utmost delicacy towards the interest and character of the professional gentleman, previously connected with the family.

XV. Some general rule should be adopted, by the faculty, in every town, relative to the *pecuniary acknowledgments* of their patients; and

and it should be deemed a point of honour to adhere to this rule, with as much steadiness, as varying circumstances will admit. For it is obvious that an average fee, as suited to the general rank of patients, must be an inadequate gratuity from the rich, who often require attendance not absolutely necessary; and yet too large to be expected from that class of citizens, who would feel a reluctance in calling for assistance, without making some decent and satisfactory retribution.

But in the consideration of fees, let it ever be remembered, that though mean ones from the affluent are both unjust and degrading, yet the characteristical beneficence of the profession is inconsistent with sordid views, and avaricious rapacity. To a young physician, it is of great importance to have clear and definite ideas of the ends of his profession; of the means for their attainment; and of the comparative value and dignity of each. Wealth, rank, and independence, with all the benefits resulting from them, are the primary ends which he holds in view; and they are interesting, wise, and laudable. But knowledge, benevolence, and active virtue, the means to be adopted in their acquisition, are of still higher estimation. And he has the privilege and felicity

licity of practising an art, even more intrinsically excellent in its mediate than in its ultimate objects. The former, therefore, have a claim to uniform pre-eminence. (k)

XVI. All members of the profession, including apothecaries as well as physicians and surgeons, together with their wives and children, should be attended *gratuitously* by any one or more of the faculty, residing near them, whose assistance may be required. For as solicitude obscures the judgment, and is accompanied with timidity and irresolution, medical men, under the pressure of sickness, either as affecting themselves or their families, are peculiarly dependent upon each other. But visits should not be obtruded officiously; as such unasked civility may give rise to embarrassment, or interfere with that choice, on which confidence depends. Distant members of the faculty, when they request attendance, should be expected to defray the charges of travelling. And if their circumstances be affluent, a pecuniary acknowledgment should not be declined: For no obligation ought to be imposed, which the party would rather compensate than contract.

 XVII. When

(k) See Notes and Illustrations, No. XI.

XVII. When a physician attends the wife or child of a member of the faculty, or any person very nearly connected with him, he should manifest peculiar attention to his opinions, and tenderness even to his prejudices. For the dear and important interests which the one has at stake, supersede every consideration of rank or seniority in the other; since the mind of a husband, a father, or a friend, may receive a deep and lasting wound, if the disease terminate fatally, from the adoption of means he could not approve, or the rejection of those he wished to be tried. Under such delicate circumstances, however, a conscientious physician will not lightly sacrifice his judgment; but will urge, with proper confidence, the measures he deems to be expedient, before he leaves the final decision concerning them to his more responsible coadjutor.

XVIII. Clergymen, who experience the *res angusta domi*, should be visited gratuitously by the faculty. And this exemption should be an acknowledged general rule, that the feeling of individual obligation may be rendered less oppressive. But such of the clergy as are qualified, either from their stipends or fortunes, to make a reasonable remuneration for medical attendance,

attendance, are not more privileged than any other order of patients. Military or naval subaltern officers, in narrow circumstances, are also proper objects of professional liberality.

XIX. As the first *consultation* by *letter* imposes much more trouble and attention than a personal visit, it is reasonable, on such an occasion, to expect a gratuity of double the usual amount. And this has long been the established practice of many respectable physicians. But a subsequent epistolary correspondence, on the further treatment of the same disorder, may justly be regarded in the light of ordinary attendance, and may be compensated, as such, according to the circumstances of the case, or of the patient.

XX. Physicians and surgeons are occasionally requested to furnish certificates, justifying the absence of persons who hold situations of honour and trust in the army, the navy, or the civil departments of government. These testimonials, unless under particular circumstances, should be considered as acts due to the public, and therefore not to be compenstaed by any gratuity. But they should never be given without an accurate and faithful scrutiny into the case; that truth and probity may not be violated, nor the good of the community injured, by the unjust pretences of its servants. The same conduct is to be observed by medical practitioners, when they are solicited to furnish apologies for non-attendance on juries; or to state the valetudinary incapacity of persons appointed to execute the business of constables, church-wardens, or overseers of the poor. No fear of giving umbrage, no view to present or future emolument, nor any motives of friendship, should incite to a false, or even dubious declaration. For the general weal requires that every individual, who is properly qualified, should deem himself obliged to execute, when legally called upon, the juridical and municipal employments of the body politic. And to be accessory, by untruth or prevarication, to the evasion of this duty, is at once a high misdemeanor against social order, and a breach of moral and professional honour.

XXI. The use of *quack medicines* should be discouraged by the faculty, as disgraceful to the profession, injurious to health, and often destructive even of life. Patients, however, under lingering disorders, are sometimes obstinately bent on having recourse to such as they see advertised, or hear recommended, with a boldness and confidence, which no intelligent physician

physician dares to adopt with respect to the means that he prescribes. In these cases, some indulgence seems to be required to a credulity that is insurmountable: And the patient should neither incur the displeasure of the physician, nor be entirely deserted by him. He may be apprized of the fallacy of his expectations, whilst assured, at the same time, that diligent attention should be paid to the process of the experiment he is so unadvisedly making on himself, and the consequent mischiefs, if any, obviated as timely as possible. Certain active preparations, the nature, composition, and effects of which are well known, ought not to be proscribed as quack medicines.

XXII. No physician or surgeon should dispense a secret *nostrum*, whether it be his invention, or exclusive property. For if it be of real efficacy, the concealment of it is inconsistent with beneficence and professional liberality. And if mystery alone give it value and importance, such craft implies either disgraceful ignorance, or fraudulent avarice.

XXIII. The *Esprit du Corps* is a principle of action founded in human nature, and when duly regulated, is both rational and laudable. Every man who enters into a fraternity engages, by a tacit compact, not only to submit

to

to the laws, but to promote the honour and interest of the association, so far as they are consistent with morality, and the general good of mankind. A physician, therefore, should cautiously guard against whatever may injure the general respectability of his profession; and should avoid all contumelious representations of the faculty at large; all general charges against their selfishness or improbity; and the indulgence of an affected or jocular scepticism, concerning the efficacy and utility of the healing art.

XXIV. As diversity of opinion and opposition of interest may in the medical, as in other professions, sometimes occasion *controversy*, and even *contention;* whenever such cases unfortunately occur, and cannot be immediately terminated, they should be referred to the arbitration of a sufficient number of physicians or of surgeons, according to the nature of the dispute; or to the two orders collectively, if belonging both to medicine and surgery. But neither the subject matter of such references, nor the adjudication, should be communicated to the public; as they may be personally injurious to the individuals concerned, and can hardly fail to hurt the general credit of the faculty.

XXV. A wealthy

XXV. A wealthy physician should not give advice *gratis* to the affluent; because it is an injury to his professional brethren. The office of physician can never be supported but as a lucrative one; and it is defrauding, in some degree, the common funds for its support, when fees are dispensed with, which might justly be claimed.

XXVI. It frequently happens that a physician, in his incidental communications with the patients of other physicians, or with their friends, may have their cases stated to him in so direct a manner, as not to admit of his declining to pay attention to them. Under such circumstances, his observations should be delivered with the most delicate propriety and reserve. He should not interfere in the curative plans pursued; and should even recommend a steady adherence to them, if they appear to merit approbation.

XXVII. A physician, when visiting a sick person in the country, may be desired to see a neighbouring patient, who is under the regular direction of another physician, in consequence of some sudden change or aggravation of symptoms. The conduct to be pursued, on such an occasion, is to give advice adapted to present circumstances; to interfere no farther than is absolutely

absolutely necessary with the general plan of treatment; to assume no future direction, unless it be expressly desired; and, in this case, to request an immediate consultation with the practitioner antecedently employed.

XXVIII. At the close of every interesting and important case, especially when it hath terminated fatally, a physician should trace back, in calm reflection, all the steps which he had taken in the treatment of it. This review of the origin, progress, and conclusion of the malady; of the whole curative plan pursued; and of the particular operation of the several remedies employed, as well as of the doses and periods of time in which they were administered, will furnish the most authentic documents, on which individual experience can be formed. But it is in a moral view that the practice is here recommended; and it should be performed with the most scrupulous impartiality. Let no self-deception be permitted in the retrospect; and if errors, either of omission or commission, are discocovered, it behoves that they should be brought fairly and fully to the mental view. Regrets may follow, but criminality will thus be obviated. For good intentions, and the imperfection of human skill which cannot anticipate the knowledge that events alone disclose, will sufficiently justify what is past, provided the failure be màde conscientiously subservient to future wisdom and rectitude in professional conduct.

XXIX. The opportunities, which a physician not unfrequently enjoys, of promoting and strengthening the good resolutions of his patients, suffering under the consequences of vicious conduct, ought never to be neglected. And his councils, or even remonstrances, will give satisfaction, not disgust, if they be conducted with politeness; and evince a genuine love of virtue, accompanied by a sincere interest in the welfare of the person to whom they are addressed.

XXX. The observance of the sabbath is a duty to which medical men are bound, so far as is compatible with the urgency of the cases under their charge. Visits may often be made with sufficient convenience and benefit, either before the hours of going to church, or during the intervals of public worship. And in many chronic ailments, the sick, together with their attendants, are qualified to participate in the social offices of religion; and should not be induced to forego this important privilege, by the expectation of a call from their physician or surgeon. *(l)*

XXXI. A physician who is advancing in years, yet unconscious of any decay in his faculties, may occasionally experience some change in the wonted confidence of his friends. Patients, who before trusted solely to his care and skill, may now request that he will join in consultation, perhaps with a younger coadjutor. It behoves him to admit this change without dissatisfaction or fastidiousness, regarding it as no mark of disrespect; but as the exercise of a just and reasonable privilege in those by whom he is employed. The junior practitioner may well be supposed to have more ardour, than he possesses, in the treatment of diseases; to be bolder in the exhibition of new medicines; and disposed to administer old ones in doses of greater efficacy. And this union of enterprize with caution, and of fervour with coolness, may promote the successful management of a difficult and protracted case. Let the medical parties, therefore, be studious to conduct themselves towards each other with candour and impartiality; co-operating, by mutual

(l) See Notes and Illustrations, No. XII.

mutual concessions, in the benevolent discharge of professional duty. *(m)*

XXXII. The commencement of that period of senescence, when it becomes incumbent on a physician to decline the offices of his profession, it is not easy to ascertain; and the decision on so nice a point must be left to the moral discretion of the individual. For, one grown old in the useful and honourable exercise of the healing art, may continue to enjoy, and justly to enjoy, the unabated confidence of the public. And whilst exempt, in a considerable degree, from the privations and infirmities of age, he is under indispensable obligations to apply his knowledge and experience, in the most efficient way, to the benefit of mankind. For the possession of powers is a clear indication of the will of our Creator, concerning their practical direction. But in the ordinary course of nature, the bodily and mental vigour must be expected to decay progressively, though perhaps slowly, after the meridian of life is past. As age advances, therefore, a physician should, from time to time, scrutinize impartially the state of his faculties; that he may determine, *bona fide*, the precise degree in which

(m) See Notes and Illustrations. No. XIII.

which he is qualified to execute the active and multifarious offices of his profession. And whenever he becomes conscious that his memory presents to him, with faintness, those analogies, on which medical reasoning and the treatment of diseases are founded; that diffidence of the measures to be pursued perplexes his judgment; that, from a deficiency in the acuteness of his senses, he finds himself less able to distinguish signs, or to prognosticate events; he should at once resolve, though others perceive not the changes which have taken place, to sacrifice every consideration of fame or fortune, and to retire from the engagements of business. To the surgeon under similar circumstances, this rule of conduct is still more necessary. For the energy of the understanding often subsists much longer than the quickness of eye-sight, delicacy of touch, and steadiness of hand, which are essential to the skilful performance of operations. Let both the physician and surgeon never forget, that their professions are public trusts, properly rendered lucrative whilst they fulfil them; but which they are bound, by honour and probity, to relinquish, as soon as they find themselves unequal to their adequate and faithful execution. *(n)*

CHAP.

(n) See Notes and Illuſtrations, No. XIV.

CHAPTER III.

OF THE CONDUCT OF PHYSICIANS TOWARDS APOTHECARIES.

I. In the present state of physic, in this country, where the profession is properly divided into three distinct branches, a connection peculiarly intimate subsists between the physician and the apothecary; and various obligations necessarily result from it. On the knowledge, skill, and fidelity of the apothecary depend, in a very considerable degree, the reputation, the success, and usefulness of the physician. As these qualities, therefore, justly claim his attention and encouragement, the possessor of them merits his respect and patronage.

II. The apothecary is, in almost every instance, the præcursor of the physician; and being acquainted with the rise and progress of the disease, with the hereditary constitution, habits, and disposition of the patient, he may furnish very important information. It is in general, therefore, expedient, and when health or life are at stake, expediency becomes a moral duty,

duty, to confer with the apothecary, before any decisive plan of treatment is adopted; to hear his account of the malady, of the remedies which have been administered, of the effects produced by them, and of his whole experience concerning the *juvantia* and *lædentia* in the case. Nor should the future attendance of the apothecary be superseded by the physician: For if he be a man of honour, judgment, and propriety of behaviour, he will be a most valuable auxiliary through the whole course of the disorder, by his attention to varying symptoms; by the enforcement of medical directions; by obviating misapprehensions in the patient, or his family; by strengthening the authority of the physician; and by being at all times an easy and friendly medium of communication. To subserve these important purposes, the physician should occasionally make his visits in conjunction with the apothecary, and regulate by circumstances the frequency of such interviews: For if they be often repeated, little substantial aid can be expected from the apothecary, because he will have no intelligence to offer which does not fall under the observation of the physician himself; nor any opportunity of executing his *peculiar* trust, with-

out

out becoming burthensome to the patient by multiplied calls, and unseasonable assiduity.

III. This amicable *intercourse* and *co-operation* of the physician and apothecary, if conducted with the *decorum* and attention to *etiquette*, which should always be steadily observed by professional men, will add to the authority of the one, to the respectability of the other, and to the usefulness of both. The patient will find himself the object of watchful and unremitting care, and will experience that he is connected with his physician, not only personally, but by a sedulous representative and coadjutor. The apothecary will regard the free communication of the physician as a privilege and mean of improvement; he will have a deeper interest in the success of the curative plans pursued; and his honour and reputation will be directly involved in the purity and excellence of the medicines dispensed, and in the skill and care with which they are compounded.

IV. The duty and responsibility of the physician, however, are so intimately connected with these points, that no dependence on the probity of the apothecary should prevent the occasional inspection of the drugs, which he prescribes. In London, the law not only authorizes,

authorizes, but enjoins a stated examination of the simple and compound medicines kept in the shops. And the policy that is just and reasonable in the metropolis, must be proportionally so in every provincial town, throughout the kingdom. Nor will any respectable apothecary object to this necessary office, when performed with delicacy, and at seasonable times; since his reputation and emolument will be increased by it, probably in the exact *ratio*, thus ascertained, of professional merit and integrity.

V. A physician called to visit a patient in the country, should not only be *minute* in his *directions*, but should *communicate* to the apothecary the *particular view*, which he takes of the *case*; that the indications of cure may be afterwards pursued with precision and steadiness; and that the apothecary may use the discretionary power committed to him, with as little deviation as possible from the general plan prescribed. To so valuable a class of men as the country apothecaries, great attention and respect is due. And as they are the guardians of health through large districts, no opportunities should be neglected of promoting their improvement, or contributing to their stock of knowledge, either by the loan of books, the direction

direction of their studies, or by unreserved information on medical subjects. When such occasions present themselves, the maxim of our judicious poet is strictly true, "The worst avarice is that of sense." For practical improvements usually originate in towns, and often remain unknown or disregarded in situations, where gentlemen of the faculty have little intercourse, and where sufficient authority is wanting to sanction innovation.

VI. It has been observed, by a political and moral writer of great authority, that "apothe-"caries' profit is become a bye-word, denoting "something uncommonly extravagant. This "great apparent profit, however, is frequently "no more than the reasonable wages of labour. "The skill of an apothecary is a much nicer "and more delicate matter than that of any ar-"tificer whatever; and the trust which is re-"posed in him is of much greater importance. "He is the physician of the poor in all cases, "and of the rich when the distress or danger is "not very great. His reward, therefore, ought "to be suitable to his skill and his trust, and it "arises generally from the price at which he "sells his drugs. But the whole drugs which "the best employed apothecary, in a large "market town, will sell in a year, may not

" perhaps cost him above thirty or forty pounds. " Though he should sell them, therefore, for " three or four hundred, or a thousand per cent. " profit, this may frequently be no more " than the reasonable wages of his labour " charged, in the only way in which he can " charge them, upon the price of his drugs."* The statement here given exceeds the emoluments of the generality of apothecaries, in country districts. And a physician, who knows the education, skill, and persevering attention, as well as the sacrifice of ease, health, and sometimes even of life, which this profession requires, should regard it as a duty not to withdraw, from those who exercise it, any sources of reasonable profit, or the honourable means of advancement in fortune. Two practices prevail in some places injurious to the interest of this branch of the faculty, and which ought to be discouraged. One consists in suffering prescriptions to be sent to the druggist, for the sake of a small saving in expence: The other in receiving an annual stipend, usually degrading in its amount, and in the services it imposes, for being consulted on the slighter indispositions to which all families

* See Smith's Wealth of Nations, book I. chap. x.

lies are incident, and which properly fall within the province of the apothecary.

VII. Physicians are sometimes requested to visit the patients of the apothecary, in his absence. Compliance, in such cases, should always be refused, when it is likely to interfere with the consultation of the medical gentleman ordinarily employed by the sick person, or his family. Indeed this practice is so liable to abuse, and requires, in its exercise, so much caution and delicacy, that it would be for the interest and honour of the faculty to have it altogether interdicted. Physicians are the only proper substitutes for physicians; surgeons for surgeons; and apothecaries for apothecaries.

VIII. When the aid of a physician is required, the apothecary to the family is frequently called upon to recommend one. It will then behove him to learn fully whether the patient or his friends have any preference or partiality; and this he ought to consult, if it lead not to an improper choice. For the maxim of Celsus is strictly applicable, on such an occasion; *Ubi par scientia, melior est amicus medicus quam extraneus.* But if the parties concerned be entirely indifferent, the apothecary is bound to decide according to his best judgment, with a conscientious and exclusive

 regard

regard to the good of the person, for whom he is commissioned to act. It is not even sufficient that he selects the person on whom, in sickness, he reposes his own trust; for in this case friendship justly gives preponderancy; because it may be supposed to excite a degree of zeal and attention, which might overbalance superior science or abilities. Without favour or regard to any personal, family, or professional connections, he should recommend the physician whom he conscientiously believes, all circumstances considered, to be best qualified to accomplish the recovery of the patient.

IX. In the county of Norfolk, and in the city of London, benevolent institutions have been lately formed, for providing funds to relieve the widows and children of apothecaries, and occasionally also members of the profession who become indigent. Such schemes merit the sanction and encouragement of every liberal physician and surgeon. And were they thus extended, their usefulness would be greatly increased, and their permanency almost with certainty secured. Medical subscribers, from every part of Great-Britain, should be admitted, if they offer satisfactory testimonials of their qualifications. One comprehensive establishment

ment seems to be more eligible than many on a smaller scale. For it would be conducted with superior dignity, regularity, and efficiency; with fewer obstacles from interest, prejudice, or rivalship; with considerable saving in the aggregate of time, trouble, and expence; with more accuracy in the calculations relative to its funds, and consequently with the utmost practicable extension of its dividends.

CHAPTER IV.

OF PROFESSIONAL DUTIES, IN CERTAIN CASES WHICH REQUIRE A KNOWLEDGE OF LAW.

I. Gentlemen of the faculty of physic, by the authority of different parliamentary statutes, enjoy an exemption from serving on inquests or juries; from bearing armour; from being constables or church-wardens; and from all burdensome offices, whether leet or parochial. These privileges are founded on reasons highly honourable to medical men; and should operate as incentives to that diligent and assiduous discharge of professional duty, which the legislature has generously presumed to occupy the the time, and to employ the talents of physicians

cians and surgeons, in some of the most important interests of their fellow-citizens. It is perhaps on account of their being thus excused from many civil functions, that Sir William Blackstone, in his learned Commentaries, judges the study of the law to be less essential to them, than to any other class of men. He observes, that "there is no special reason why gentlemen "of the faculty of physic should apply them- "selves to the study of the law, unless in com- "mon with other gentlemen, and to complete "the character of general and extensive know- "ledge, which this profession, beyond others, "has remarkably deserved."* But I apprehend it will be found that physicians and surgeons are often called upon to exercise appropriate duties, which require not only a knowledge of the principles of jurisprudence, but of the forms and regulations adopted in our courts of judicature. The truth of this observation will sufficiently appear from the following *brief detail* of some of the principal cases, in which the science of law is of importance to medical practitioners. To enter at large on so comprehensive a subject, would far exceed the bounds of the present undertaking.

II. When

* Vol. I. sect. I. introduction.

II. When a physician attends upon a patient, under circumstances of imminent danger, his counsel may be required about the expediency of a *last will* and *testament.* It behoves him, therefore, to know whether, in case of intestacy, the daughters, or younger children of the sick person would be legally entitled to any share of his fortune: Whether the fortune would be equally divided, when such equality would be improper or unjust: Whether diversity of claims and expensive litigations would ensue, without a will, from the nature of the property in question: And whether the creditors of the defunct would, by his neglect, be defrauded of their equitable claims. For it is a culpable deficiency in our laws, that real estates are not subject to the payment of debts by simple contract, unless expressly charged with them by the last will and testament of the proprietor; although credit is often founded, as Dr. Paley well observes, on the possession of such estates. This acute moralist adds, "He, therefore, who neglects to make the necessary appointments for "the payment of his debts, as far as his effects "extend, sins in his grave; and if he omits "this on purpose to defeat the demands of his "creditors,

"creditors, he dies with a deliberate fraud in "his heart."*

Property is divided by the law into two species, *personal* and *real;* each requiring appropriate modes of transfer or alienation, with which a physician should be well acquainted. It may also be required of him to deliver an opinion, and even a solemn judicial evidence, concerning the *capacity* of his patient to make a *will*, a point sometimes of difficult and nice decision. For various disorders obscure, without perverting, the intellectual faculties. And even in delirium itself there are lucid intervals, when the memory and judgment become sufficiently clear, accurate, and vigorous, for the valid execution of a testament. In such cases the will should commence with the signature of the testator, concluding with it also, if his hand be not, after continued mental exertions, too tremulous for subscription; and it should be made with all possible conciseness, and expedition.†

If

* See Paley's Principles of Moral and Political Philosophy, book III. part I. chap. xxiii.

† "In the construction of the statute, 29 Car. II. c. 3. "it has been adjudged that the testator's name, written "with

If the patient be surprized by sudden and violent sickness, the law authorizes a *nuncupative will* in the disposal of personalty. But to guard against fraud, the testamentary words must be delivered with an explicit intention to bequeath; the will must be made at home, or among the testator's family and friends, unless by unavoidable accident; and also in his last sickness: For if he recover, it is evident that time is given for a written will.*

The law excludes from the privilege of making a will *madmen, ideots,* persons in their *dotage,* or those who have stupefied their understandings by drunkenness. But there is a high degree of hypochondriacism, which not unfrequently falls under the cognizance of a physician, and on which he may be required to decide whether it amounts to mental incapacity for the execution of a last will and testament. To define the precise boundaries of rationality is perhaps impossible; if it be true, according to Shakespear, that " the lunatic, the lover, and the

 poet

" with his own hand, at the beginning of the will, as I, " John Mills, do make this my last will and testament; " is a sufficient signing, without any name at the bottom, " though the other is the safer way." See Blackstone's Comment. Book II. chap. xxiii.

* Id. Book II. c. 32.

poet are of imagination all compact." But a partially distempered fancy is known to subsist with general intelligence: And a man, like Mr. Simon Browne, believing the extinction of his rational soul by the judgment of God, may uniformly evince, in every other instance, very distinguished intellectual powers; and be capable of directing his concerns, and disposing of his property, with sufficient discretion. To preclude one, so affected, from being a testator, seems inconsistent either with wisdom or justice; especially if the will, which has been made, discover, in its essential parts, no traces of a disturbed imagination or unsound judgment. But whenever false ideas, of a *practical kind*, are so firmly united as to be constantly and invariably mistaken for truth, we properly denominate this unnatural alliance INSANITY. And if it give rise to a train of subordinate wrong associations, producing incongruity of behaviour, incapacity for the common duties of life, or unconscious deviations from morality and religion, MADNESS has then its commencement. *(o)*

III. A lunatic,

(o) See the Author's Moral and Literary Dissertations, p. 127, second edit.;—also Notes and Illustrations, No. XV.

III. A lunatic, or *non compos mentis*, in the eye of the law, is one who has had understanding, but has lost it by disease, grief, or other accident. The king is the trustee for such unfortunate persons, appointed to protect their property, and to account to them, if they recover, for their revenues; or, after their decease, to their representatives. The Lord Chancellor, therefore, grants a commission to inquire into the state of mind of the insane person; and if he be found *non compos*, he usually commits the care of his person, with a suitable allowance for his maintenance, to some friend, who is then called his committee.* The physician, who has been consulted about the case, will doubtless be called upon to deliver an opinion concerning his patient. And before he becomes accessory to his deprivation, as it were, of all legal existence, he will weigh attentively the whole circumstances of the disorder; the original cause of it; the degree in which it subsists; its duration, and probable continuance. For if the malady be not fixed, great, and permanent, this solemn act of law must be deemed inexpedient, because it cannot be reversed without difficulty. And when insanity

 has

* Blackstone's Comment. Book I. chap. viii.

has been once formally declared, there may be grounds of apprehension that the party will be consigned to neglect and oblivion. With regard to the waste or alienation of property by the person thus afflicted, little risque is incurred, if he be put under the ordinary restraint of a judicious *curator*. For whilst his mind remains in the state of alienation, he is incapable of executing any act with validity; and the next heir, or other person interested, may set it aside, on the plea of his incapacity. But the use of a guardian or committee of a lunatic is chiefly to renew, in his right, under the direction of the court of chancery, any lease for lives or years, and to apply the profits for the benefit of the insane person, of his heirs, or executors.

IV. The law justifies the *beating of a lunatic, in such manner as the circumstances may require.** But it has been before remarked that a physician, who attends an asylum for insanity, is under an obligation of honour as well as of humanity, to secure to the unhappy sufferers, committed to his charge, all the tenderness and indulgence compatible with steady and effectual government.

* I. Hawkins 130. Burn's Justice, vol. III. pag. 117.

government.* And the strait waistcoat, with other improvements in modern practice, now preclude the necessity of coercion by corporal punishment.

V. Houses for the reception of lunatics are subject to strict regulations of law. These regulations refer to the persons keeping such houses, to the admission of patients into them, and to their inspection by visitors, duly authorized and qualified. If any one conceal more than a single lunatic without a licence, he becomes liable to a penalty of five hundred pounds. The licences in the cities of London and Westminster, or within seven miles of the metropolis, are granted by the college of physicians; who are empowered to elect five of their fellows to act as commissioners for inspecting the lunatic asylums, within their jurisdiction. Houses for the reception of lunatics in the country, are to be licenced by the justices of the peace, during their quarter sessions: And at the time when the licence is granted, the magistrates are directed to nominate two of their own body, and also one physician, to visit and inspect such licensed houses. This inspection they are empowered to make as often as

* Chap II. Sect. XXX.

as they judge it to be expedient; and an allowance is to be granted for the expences incurred. The keeper of every licensed house is bound, under the penalty of one hundred pounds, not to admit or confine any person as a lunatic, without having a certificate in writing, under the hand and seal of some physician, surgeon, or apothecary, that such person is proper to be received into the house, as being *non compos mentis*. And he is further required, under the same penalty, to give notice of this certificate to the secretary of the commissioners, appointed either by the college of physicians, or the magistrates at their quarter-sessions. The act of parliament, which establishes these regulations, states this important proviso, "That in all proceedings which shall be had under his Majesty's writ of *Habeas Corpus*, and in all indictments, informations, and actions, that shall be preferred or brought against any person or persons for confining or ill-treating any of his Majesty's subjects, in any of the said houses, the parties complained of shall be obliged to justify their proceedings according to the course of the common law, in the same manner as if this act had not been made."*

The

* See Statutes at Large, Vol. VIII. 14 Geo. III. C. 49.

The legal allowance to a medical commissioner, for the visitation and inspection of a lunatic-asylum, is fixed, by the statute, at one guinea. This gratuity, which cannot be regarded as a just compensation for the time and trouble bestowed, it may often be proper to decline. For to a physician, of a liberal mind, an inadequate pecuniary acknowledgment is felt as a degradation; but he will be amply remunerated by the consciousness of having performed an office, enjoined at once by the laws of humanity, and of his country.

VI. In the case of *sudden death*, the law has made provision for examining into the cause of it, by the *Coroner*, an officer appointed for the purpose, who is empowered to summon such evidence as is necessary, for the discharge of his inquisitorial and judicial functions. On these occasions, the attendance of a physician or surgeon may often be required, who should be qualified to give testimony consonant to legal, as well as to medical knowledge. To this end, he must not only be acquainted with the signs of natural death, but also of those which occur, when it is produced by accident or violence. And he should not be a stranger to the several distinctions of homicide, established in our courts of judicature. For the division of this

this act into *justifiable*, *excusable*, and *felonious*, will aid his investigation, and give precision to the opinion which he delivers.

VII. When a crime, which the law has adjudged to be capital, is attempted to be committed by force, the resistance of such force, even so as to occasion the death of the offender, is deemed *justifiable homicide*. Mr. Locke, in his Essay on Government, carries this doctrine to a much greater extent; asserting, that "all manner of force, without a right, upon a "man's person, puts him in a state of war with "the aggressor, and of consequence, being in "such a state of war, he may lawfully kill him "that puts him under this unnatural restraint."* But Judge Blackstone considers this conclusion as applicable only to a state of uncivilized nature; and observes, that the law of England is too tender of the public peace, too careful of the life of the subject, to adopt so contentious a system; nor will suffer, with impunity, any crime to be *prevented* by death, unless the same, if committed, would also be punished by death.†

VIII. With

* Essay on Government, Part II. ch. iii.

† Blackstone's Comment. Book IV. ch. xiv.

VIII. With cases of justifiable homicide, however, gentlemen of the faculty are seldom likely to be professionally concerned. But *excusable homicide* may frequently fall under their cognizance, and require their deliberate attention, and accurate investigation. It is of two sorts; either *per infortunium*, by misadventure; or *se defendendo*, upon a principle of self-preservation. Death may be the consequence of a lawful act, done without any intention of hurt. Thus if an officer, in the correction of a soldier by the sentence of a court martial, happen to occasion his death, it is only misadventure; the punishment being lawful. But if the correction be unwarrantably severe, either in the manner, the instrument, or the duration of punishment, and death ensue, the offender is at least guilty of manslaughter, and in some circumstances, of murder. A surgeon, therefore, is usually present, when soldiers are chastized with the lash; and on his testimony must depend the justification of the mode and degree of punishment inflicted.—When medicines administered to a sick patient, with an honest design, to produce the alleviation of his pain, or cure of his disease, occasion death, this is misadventure, in the view of the law; and the physician or surgeon, who directed them, is not liable to punishment criminally, though a civil action might formerly lie for neglect or ignorance. But it hath been holden that such immunity is confined to *regular* physicians and surgeons. Sir Matthew Hale, however, justly questions the legality of this determination; since physic and salves were in use before licensed physicians and surgeons. "Wherefore he treats the doctrine "as apocryphal, and fitted only to qualify and "flatter licenciates and doctors in physic; "though it may be of use to make people "cautious how they meddle too much in so "dangerous an employment." The college of physicians, however, within their jurisdiction, which extends seven miles round London, are vested by charter with the power of fine and imprisonment *pro mala praxi*. Yet Dr. Groenvelt, who was cited, in the year 1693, before the Censors of the College, and committed to Newgate, by a warrant from the president, for prescribing *cantharides* in substance, was acquitted on the plea that bad practice must be accompanied with a bad intention, to render it criminal. This prosecution, whilst it ruined the doctor's reputation, and injured his fortune, so that he is said to have died in want, excited general attention to the remedy, and afterwards established

established the use of it; though it must be acknowledged that his doses were too bold and hazardous. But whatever be the indulgence of the law towards medical practitioners, they are bound by a higher authority than that of the most solemn statute, not to exercise the healing art without due knowledge, tenderness, and discretion: And every rash experiment, every mistake originating from gross inattention, or from that ignorance which necessarily results from defective education, is, in the eye of conscience, a crime both against God and man.

It must frequently devolve on the faculty to decide concerning the nature and effects of blows, strokes, or wounds inflicted, and how far the death of the sufferer is to be ascribed to them, or to some antecedent or subsequent disease. In homicide, also, *se defendendo*, the manner and time of the defence are to be considered. For if the person assaulted fall upon the aggressor, when the fray is over and he is running away, this is revenge and not defence. And though no witness were present, the situation of the wound or of the blow would afford, if in the back of the assailant, presumptive evidence of *felonious homicide*.

IX. This crime, which in atrocity exceeds every other, is considered by the law under the three heads of *suicide*, *manslaughter*, and *murder*, concerning each of which the faculty are occasionally obliged to give professional evidence. A *felo de se* is one who has deliberately put an end to his existence, or committed any unlawful malicious act, the immediate consequence of which proved death to himself. To constitute this act a crime, the party must have been of years of discretion, and in the possession of reason. A physician, therefore, may be called upon, by the coroner, to state his opinion of the mental capacity of the defunct. And the law will not authorise the plea, that every melancholic or hypochondriac fit deprives a man of the power of discerning right from wrong. Even if a lunatic kill himself in a lucid interval, Sir M. Hale affirms that he is a *felo de se*.— And the physician, who has attended him, is best qualified to judge of the degree, the duration, or periodical seasons of such returns of sanity. But there are cases of temporary distraction, when death may be rushed upon apparently with design, but really from the influence of terror, or the want of that presence of mind, which is necessary to the exercise of judgment, and the discrimination of actual from imaginary evil. Of this kind the reader will find an affecting instance, related by by Dr. Hunter, in the Medical Observations and Inquiries, published by a Society of Physicians in London.*

X. *Manslaughter* is defined "the unlawful "killing of another, without malice, express "or implied; which may be either *voluntarily*, "upon a sudden heat; or *involuntarily*, but in "the commission of some unlawful act." Yet though this definition is delivered from Sir Matthew Hale, by the excellent commentator on the laws of England so often quoted, it is not sufficiently precise and comprehensive. For when a person does an act lawful in itself, but which proves fatal to a fellow-citizen, because done without due circumspection, it may, according to circumstances, be either misadventure, manslaughter, or murder. Thus when a workman kills any one, by flinging down a stone or piece of timber into the street, if the accident be in a country village, where there are few passengers, and if he give warning by calling out to them, it is only misadventure: But if it be in London, or any other populous town, where persons are continually passing, it is manslaughter, though warning be loudly given: And it is murder, if he know of their passing,

* Vol. VI. p. 279.

passing, and yet gives no warning; for this is malice against all mankind.*

On the like grounds we may reason concerning the cases of death, occasioned by drugs designed to produce abortion. This purpose is not always unlawful: For the configuration of the *pelvis*, in some females, is such as to render the birth of a full grown child impossible, or inevitably fatal. But even in such instances, the guilt manslaughter may be incurred by ignorance of the drastic quality of the medicine prescribed, or want of due caution in the dose administered. And when no moral or salutary end is in view, the simple act itself, if fatal in the issue, falls under the denomination of murder.† "If a woman "be quick with child, and, by a potion or otherwise, killeth it in her womb, this is a great "misprision, yet no murder: But if the child "be born alive, and dieth of the potion or "other cause, this is murder."‡ The procuring of abortions was common amongst the Romans; and, it is said, was liable to no penalty, before the reigns of Severus and Antoninus. Even those princes made it criminal only in the case of a married woman, practising it to defraud

* Blackstone's Comment. Book IV. ch. xiv.

† See Burn's Justice of Peace, vol. I. p. 216.

‡ Id. vol. II. p. 110.

defraud her husband of the comforts of children, from motives of resentment. For the *fœtus* being regarded as a portion of the womb of the mother, she was supposed to have an equal and full right over both. This false opinion may have its influence in modern, as well as in ancient times; and false it must be deemed, since no female can be privileged to injure her own bowels, much less the *fœtus*, which is now well known to constitute no part of them. To extinguish the first spark of life is a crime of the same nature, both against our Maker and society, as to destroy an infant, a child, or a man; these regular and successive stages of existence being the ordinances of God, subject alone to his divine will, and appointed by sovereign wisdom and goodness as the exclusive means of preserving the race, and multiplying the enjoyments of mankind. Hence the father of physic, in the oath enjoined on his pupils, which some universities now impose on the candidates for medical degrees, obliged them solemnly to abjure the practice of administering the πεσσος φθοριος. But in weighing the charge, against any person, of having procured abortion, the methods employed should be attentively considered by the faculty; as this effect has often been ascribed to causes inadequate to its production.

production. Even the pessary, so sanctimoniously forbidden by Hippocrates, has little of that activity and power, which superstition assigned to it.

XI. The law of England guards, with assiduous care, the lives of infants, when endangered by motives which counteract, and too often overbalance, the strong operation of maternal love. In cases of *bastardy*, therefore, it is declared, by a statute passed in the reign of James the first, that "If any woman "be delivered of any issue of her body, male "or female, which being born alive, should by "the laws of this realm be a bastard, and she "endeavour privately, either by drowning, or "secret burying thereof, or any other way, "either by herself, or the procuring of others, "so to conceal the death thereof, as that it "may not come to light whether it was born "alive or not, but be concealed, she shall suffer "death, as in case of murder, except she can "prove, by one witness at least, that the child "was born dead."* This law, though humane in its principle, is much too severe in its construction. To give certainty to punishment, by facilitating conviction, is doubtless an essential object

* Burn's Justice, vol. I. p. 216.

object of jurisprudence. And it has been well observed, that the statute, which made the possession of the implements of coining a capital offence, by constituting such possession complete evidence of guilt, has proved the most effectual mean of enforcing the denunciation of law against this dangerous and tempting crime.* But the analogy, which the able moralist has drawn between this ordinance and that relating to bastardy, is not fully conclusive. For possession, in the former case, clearly implies a specific purpose, for which the legislature, with sufficient wisdom and justice, has provided a specific punishment. Whereas secrecy in the mother, concerning the death of her illegitimate offspring, hardly amounts to the lowest degree of presumptive evidence of felonious homicide. Gentlemen of the faculty have often melancholy experience of the distraction and misery, which females suffer under these unhappy circumstances. And when it becomes their painful office to deliver evidence, on such occasions, justice and humanity require, that they should scrutinize the whole truth, and *nothing extenuate, nor set down aught*

* See Paley's Moral and Political Philosophy, 4to. p. 350.

in malice. "What is commonly understood to "be the murder of a bastard child by the mo- "ther," says Dr. Hunter, "if the real circum- "stances were fully known, would be allowed "to be a very different crime in different cir- "cumstances. In some (it is to be hoped "*rare*) instances, it is a crime of the very "deepest dye.......But, as well as I can judge, "the greatest number of what are called mur- "ders of bastard children, are of a very dif- "ferent kind. The mother has an unconquer- "able sense of shame, and pants after the pre- "servation of character: So far she is virtuous "and amiable. She has not the resolution to "meet and avow infamy. In proportion as "she loses the hope either of having been mis- "taken with regard to pregnancy, or of being "relieved from her terrors by a fortunate mis- "carriage, she every day sees her danger greater "and nearer, and her mind overwhelmed with "terror and despair. In this situation many of "these women, who are afterwards accused of "murder, would destroy themselves, if they "did not know that such an action would in- "fallibly lead to an inquiry, which would pro- "claim what they are so anxious to conceal. "In this perplexity, and meaning nothing less "than the murder of the infant, they are me-

"ditating

" ditating different schemes for concealing the " death of the child; but are wavering between " difficulties on all sides, putting the evil hour " off, and trusting too much to chance and for- " tune. In that state often they are overtaken " before they expected; their schemes are frus- " trated; their distress of body and mind de- " prives them of all judgment and rational con- " duct; they are delivered by themselves where- " ver they happen to retire in their fright or " confusion; sometimes dying in the agonies of " childbirth, and sometimes being quite ex- " hausted they faint away, and become insen- " sible of what is passing; and when they re- " cover a little strength, find that the child, " whether still-born or not, is completely life- " less. In such a case, is it to be expected, " when it would answer no purpose, that a " woman should divulge the secret? Will not " the best dispositions of mind urge her to " preserve her character? She will therefore " hide every appearance of what has happened " as well as she can, though if the discovery " be made, that conduct will be set down as a " proof of her guilt."...... " Here let us sup- " pose a case, which every body will allow to " be very possible. An unmarried woman, " becoming pregnant, is striving to conceal

" her shame, and laying the best scheme that " she can devise, for saving her own life and " that of the child, and at the same time con- " cealing the secret; but her plan is at once " disconcerted by her being taken ill by herself, " and delivered of a dead child. If the law " punishes such a woman with death for con- " cealing her shame, does it not require more " from human nature, than weak human na- " ture can bear? In a case so circumstanced, " surely the only crime is the having been preg- " nant, which the law does not mean to punish " with death; and the attempt to conceal it by " fair means should not be punishable with " death, as that attempt seems to arise from a " principle of virtuous shame."*

The observations, here quoted, have a just claim to attention, from the extensive experience which the author possessed, and still more from his intimate knowledge of the female character. Yet to the moral and political philosopher, Dr. Hunter may appear to have exalted the sense of shame into the principle of virtue; and to have mistaken the great end of penal law, which is not vengeance but the prevention of crimes. The statute, indeed, which

* Med. Obs. and Inq. vol. VI. p. 271. et seq.

which makes the concealment of the birth of a bastard child full proof of murder, confounds all distinctions of innocence and guilt, as such concealment, whenever practicable, would be the wish and act of all mothers, virtuous or vicious, under the same unhappy predicament. Law, however, which is the guardian and bulwark of the public weal, must maintain a steady, and even rigid watch, over the general tendencies of human actions: And when these are not only clearly understood, but interpreted according to the rules of wisdom and rectitude, that may justly be constituted a civil crime, which, if permitted, might give occasion to atrocious guilt, though in its own nature innocent. The measure of punishment, however, should be proportionate, as nearly as possible, to the temptation to offend, and to the kind and degree of evil produced by the offence. If inadequate to the former it will be nugatory; and if too severe for the latter, it will defeat itself, by furnishing a just plea for superseding its execution.* A revision of our sanguinary statutes is much wanted; and it would be happy

* "L'atrocité des lois en empêche l'exécution.

"Lorsque la peine est sans mesure, on est souvent obligé de lui préférer l'impunité."

MONTESQUIEU.

happy if means could be devised of suppressing the punishment, by obviating the crime, when it is merely positive or municipal. This we have seen accomplished with respect to the coinage of money, by the simple introduction of a standard weight in the payment of gold. And a sagacious legislator might doubtless discover and adopt similar improvements, in other branches of penal jurisprudence.

Much observation is required to discriminate between a child still born, and one that has lived after birth only a short space of time. Various appearances, also, both internal and external, may be mistaken for marks of violent death. Even the swimming of the lungs in water, a test on which so much reliance is placed, will, on many occasions, be found fallacious. But these arc points of professional science, which do not strictly fall under the subject of this section; and the reader is particularly referred to the paper already quoted, and also to the *Elementa Medicinæ Forensis Joh. Fred. Faselii;* or to a valuable epitome of the same work in English by Dr. Farr.*

XII. *Duelling*

* Elements of Medical Jurisprudence: or a succinct and compendious Description of such Tokens in the Human Body, as are requisite to determine the Judgment of

XII. *Duelling* is another species of felony, even though the consequences of it should not prove fatal: And gentlemen of the faculty are peculiarly interested in the knowledge of the laws relating to it; because they are not only liable to be summoned on the trial of the parties, if either or both of them be wounded, but are frequently professional attendants on them in the field of combat. It is astonishing that a practice, which originated in ages of Gothic ignorance, superstition, and barbarism, should be continued in the present enlightened period, though condemned by the ordinances of every state, and repugnant to the spirit and precepts of Christianity. Sir Francis Bacon, when attorney-general, in the reign of James I. delivered a charge, before the court of star-chamber, touching duels, which gives a clear and animated view of the light in which they were then regarded. "The first motive," he says, "is a false and erroneous imagination "of honour and credit; and, therefore, the "king, in his proclamation, doth most aptly "call them *bewitching duels*. For if one judge "of it truly, it is no better than a sorcery, "that

a Coroner, and of Courts of Law, in Cases of Divorce, Rape, Murder, &c. London, Becket, 1788.

"that enchanteth the spirits of young men, "and a kind of satanical illusion and apparition of honour against religion, against "law, and against moral virtue. Hereunto "may be added that men have almost lost the "true notion and understanding of fortitude "and valour. For fortitude distinguisheth of "the grounds of quarrels whether they be just; "and not only so, but whether they be worthy; "and setteth a better price upon men's lives "than to bestow them idly: Nay it is weakness "and disesteem of a man's self, to put a man's "life upon such liedger performances: A man's "life is not to be trifled away; it is to be offered up and sacrificed to honourable services, "public merits, good causes, and noble adventures. It is in expence of blood as it is in "expence of money; it is no liberality to make "a profusion of money upon every vain occasion; nor no more is it fortitude to make "effusion of blood, except the cause be of "worth."*

The decree of the Star Chamber against Priest and Wright, the objects of Sir Francis Bacon's charge, was, that they should both be committed to prison; that the former should be fined £500, and the latter 500 marks, and that

* Bacon's Works, 4to. Birch's edit. vol. II. p. 565.

that at the next assizes they should publicly acknowledge their high contempt of, and offence against God, the king's majesty, and his laws, shewing themselves penitent for the same.—Though this judgment appears to have been founded in wisdom and equity, yet, happily for our country, the court, which passed the sentence, has been long suppressed; and we are now governed not by arbitrary will, but by known and fixed laws. Those which subsist against duelling, I shall quote on the authorities of Foster, Blackstone, Hawkins, and Burn. "Deliberate duelling, if death ensueth, is in "the eye of the law, murder; for duels are generally founded in deep revenge; and though "a person should be drawn into a duel, "not upon a motive so criminal, but merely "upon the punctilio of what the swordsmen "falsely call honour, that will not excuse; for "he that deliberately seeketh the blood of another upon a private quarrel, acteth in defiance "of all laws human and divine."* "Express "malice is when one, with a sedate deliberate "mind and formed design, doth kill another. "This takes in the case of deliberate duelling, "where both parties meet, avowedly, with any

 "intent

* Sir Michael Foster's Reports, 8vo. p. 297.

" intent to murder; thinking it their duty as " gentlemen, and claiming it as their right, to " wanton with their own lives, and those of " their fellow-creatures, without any warrant " or authority from any power either human or ' divine, but in direct contradiction to the laws " both of God and man. And therefore, the " law has justly fixed the crime and punish- " ment of murder on them, and on their seconds " also.* " The law so abhors all duelling in " cold blood, that not only the principal who " actually kills the other, but also his seconds, " are guilty of murder, whether they fought or " not: And it is holden that the seconds of the " party slain are also guilty as accessaries."†— From variations in the moral and intellectual character of man, it is impossible to ascertain the precise period, when the passions may be supposed to become cool, after having been violently agitated. Judgment, therefore, must be founded on the circumstances of deliberation, which are delivered in the course of evidence. In many cases, it has been determined that death, in consequence of an appointment and meeting,

* Blackstone's Comment. Book IV. ch. xiv.

† I Hawkins 82; and Burn's Justice, vol. II. p. 509.

meeting, a few hours subsequent to the provocation, is murder.*

XIII. Before a surgeon engage professionally to *attend* a *duellist* to the *field* of *combat*, it behoves him to consider well, not only how far he is about to countenance a deliberate violation of the duties of morality and religion; but whether, in the construction of law, he may not be deemed an aider and abettor of a crime, which involves in it such turpitude, that death is alike denounced against the principal and the accessary. Does he not voluntarily put himself into a predicament, similar, in many essential points, to that of the *second*, who is expressly condemned by the legislature of this country? Both are apprized of the purpose to commit an act of felony: Both take an interest in the circumstances attendant upon it: And both are present during the execution; the one to regulate its antecedents, the other to alleviate its consequences. But I suggest these considerations with much diffidence: And though I observe some passages, in Sir Michael Foster's Discourse concerning Accomplices, which seem to confirm them; yet it may be proper to quote the following, apparently adverse, opinion of this

* See Legg's ca. Kelyng 27. Eden's Principles of Penal Law, p. 224.

this excellent judge. "In order to render a "person an accomplice and a principal in fe- "lony, he must be aiding and abetting at the "fact, or ready to afford assistance, if necessary. "And therefore if A happeneth to be present "at a murder, for instance, and taketh no "part in it, nor endeavoureth to prevent it, "nor apprehendeth the murderer, nor levieth "hue and cry after him, this strange behaviour "of his, though highly criminal, will not of "itself render him either principal or acces- "sary."*

But whatever be the objections against the attendance of a surgeon in the field of combat, they cannot be construed to extend to the affording of all possible assistance, to any unfortunate sufferer, in an affair of honour; provided such assistance be not preconcerted, but required as in ordinary accidents or emergencies. For in the offices of the healing art, no discrimination can be made, either of occasions or of characters. And it must be acknowledged, that many of the victims of duelling have been men, from their talents and virtues, possessing the justest claim to assiduous and tender attention. That lives of such inestimable value

* Foster's Crown Law, 8vo. p. 350.

lure to their friends, to their families, and to the public, should be at the mercy of any profligate rake, who wantonly gives affronts, or idly fancies he receives them, is a great aggravation of the folly, as well as of the guilt of duelling. This reflection seems to shew the propriety of a change in the penal code, respecting it; and that the punishment inflicted should be confined to the aggressor; strict inquisition into the circumstances of the case being previously made, by the coroner, or some magistrate authorized and bound to exercise this important trust. And he may, with reason, be regarded as the aggressor, who either violates the rules of decorum, by any unprovoked rudeness or insult; or who converts into an offence, what was intended only as convivial pleasantry. *(p)*

XIV. A physician has no special interest in an acquaintance with the statutes relative to duelling. But as he possesses the rank of a gentleman, both by his liberal education and profession, the *law of honour*, if that may be termed a law which is indefinite and arbitrary, has a claim to his serious study and attention. As a philosopher, also, it becomes him to trace its

(p) See Notes and Illuſtrations, No. XVII.

its origin, and to investigate the principles on which it is founded: And as a moralist, duty calls upon him to counteract its baneful influence and ascendancy. For, in principle, it is distinct from virtue; and, as a practical rule, it extends only to certain formalities and decorums, of little importance in the transactions of life, and which are spontaneously observed by those, who are actuated with the true sense of propriety and rectitude. Genuine honour, in its full extent, may be defined a quick perception and strong feeling of moral obligation, in conjunction with an acute sensibility to shame, reproach, or infamy. In different characters, these constituent parts of the principle are found to exist in proportions so diversified, as sometimes to appear almost single and detached. The former always *aids and strengthens virtue;* the latter may occasionally *imitate her actions,** when fashion happily countenances, or high example prompts to rectitude. But being connected, for the most part, with a jealous pride and capricious irritability, it will be more shocked with the *imputation,* than with the *commission* of what is wrong. And thus it will constitute that spurious honour, which,

* Addison's Cato.

which, by a perversion of the laws of association, *puts evil for good and good for evil;* and, under the sanction of a name, perpetrates crimes without remorse, and even without ignominy.*

XV. *Homicide* by *poison* is another very important object of medical jurisprudence.—When it is the effect of inadvertency, or the want of adequate caution, in the use of substances dangerous to health and life, the law regards it as a misdemeanour: When it is the consequence of rashness, of wanton experiment, or of motives unjust though not malicious,† it becomes manslaughter: And when the express purpose is to kill, by means of some deleterious drug, it constitutes a most atrocious species of murder. In cases of this nature, the

* See the Author's Mor. and Lit. Diss. p. 295. 2d. Edit.

† "If an action unlawful itself be done deliberately, "and *with intention of mischief*, or great bodily harm to par-"ticulars, or of mischief indiscriminately, fall it where "it may, and death ensue against or beside the original in-"tention of the party, it will be murder. But if such "*mischievous intention* doth not appear, which is matter of "fact and *to be collected from circumstances*, and the act "was done heedlessly and incautiously, it will be man-"slaughter; not accidental death, because the act which "ensued was unlawful." Foster, p. 261.

the faculty are called upon to give evidence concerning the nature of the poison, the symptoms produced by it, and the actual fatality of its operation. I know not whether the period of this fatal operation be extended, as in the infliction of blows and wounds, to a year and a day. But if it be, the most nice and accurate investigation of the progressive advances of disease and death will be incumbent on the physician or surgeon, who is consulted on the occasion. No subject has given rise to more misconception and superstition, than the action of poisons. Numberless substances have been classed as such, which, if not inert, are at least innoxious; and powers have been ascribed to others, far exceeding their real energy.— Even Lord Verulam, the great luminary of science, in his charge against the Earl of Somerset, for the murder of Sir Thomas Overbury, in the tower of London, seems to give credit to the story of Livia, who is said to have poisoned the figs upon the tree, which her husband was wont to gather with his own hands. And he seriously states, that "Weston "chased the poor prisoner with poison after "poison; poisoning salts, poisoning meats, "poisoning sweet-meats, poisoning medicines "and vomits, until at last his body was almost "come,

"come, by the use of poisons, to the state "that Mithridates's body was by the use of "treacle and preservatives, that the force of "the poisons was blunted upon him: Weston "confessing, when he was tried for not dis-"patching him, that he had given enough to "poison twenty men."* In this criminal transaction the truth probably was, what has been judiciously suggested by Rapin, that the lieutenant of the tower, refusing to be concerned in the crime, yet not daring to discover it, from the fear of the Viscount Rochester's resentment, seized the victuals, sent from time to time for the prisoner, and threw them into the house of office. Sir Thomas Overbury, however, fell a victim at last to an empoisoned glyster.

When the particular drug, or other mean employed, can be accurately ascertained, its deleterious qualities should be fully investigated; and these should be cautiously compared with the effects ascribed to it, in the case under consideration. It may often be expedient, also, to examine the body of the sufferer by dissection; and this should be accomplished as expeditiously as possible; that the changes

N imputed

* Bacon's Works, vol. II. p. 614.

imputed to death may not be confounded with those which are imputed to poison. But on such points reference can alone be made to the knowledge and experience of the practitioner, and to the lights which he may acquire by consulting Faselius, and other works of a similar nature. I shall, therefore, close this article with a few passages of the charge of Mr. Justice Buller to the grand jury, relative to the trial of Captain Donellan, for the murder of Sir Theodosius Boughton, at the Warwick assizes, in March 1781. "In this case, gen-"tlemen," he says, "you will have two ob-"jects to consider,' first, whether the deceased "did die of *poison?* secondly, whether the "person suspected did assist in *administering* "the poison? With respect to the first of these "considerations, you will, no doubt, *hear the* "*sentiments of those who are skilled in the na-*"*ture and effects of poison*, which is of various "sorts, and most subtile in its operation.— "From the *information* of such persons you "will be able to form an opinion of the effects "which *different poisons* have on *different* "*persons*; and also the effects the *same poisons* "have on persons of *different habits and con-*"*stitutions*. If you find he did get his death "by poison, the next case is, to consider, "who

" who gave him that poison. Where poison " is knowingly given, and death ensues, it is " wilful murder; and if one is present, when " poison is given by another, he is not an ac- " cessary but a principal."*

XVI. In all civilized countries, the honour and chastity of the female sex are guarded from violence, by the severest sanctions of law. And this protection is at once humane, just, and necessary to social morality. It is consonant to humanity that weakness should be secured against the attacks of brutal strength: It is just that the most sacred of all personal property should be preserved from invasion:— And it is essential to morality that licentious passion should be restrained; that modesty should not be wounded; nor the mind contaminated, in some instances, before it is capable of forming adequate conceptions of right and wrong. The crime of *rape*, therefore, subjects the perpetrator to condign punishment by every code of jurisprudence, ancient or modern. *(q)* Amongst the Jews death was inflicted, if the damsel were betrothed to another man: And if not betrothed, a fine, amounting to fifty she-

* Hist. Sketches of Civil Liberty, p. 209.

(q) See Notes and Illustrations, No. XVI.

kels of silver, was to be paid to her father by him who had *laid hold of the virgin*, and she was to become his wife: And because *he had humbled her, he might not put her away all his days*:* For the privilege of divorce was authorized by the Jewish institutions. The Romans made this offence capital, superadding the confiscation of goods. Even the carrying-off a woman from her parents or guardians, and cohabiting with her, whether accomplished by force, or with her full consent, were made equally penal with a rape, by an imperial edict. For the Roman law seems to have supposed, that women never deviate from virtue, without being seduced by the arts of the other sex.— And, therefore, by imposing a powerful restraint on the solicitations of men, they aimed at a more effectual security of the chastity of women. *Nisi etenim eam solicitaverit, nisi odiosis artibus circumvenerit, non faciet eam velle in tantum dedecus sese prodere.* But the English law, as Judge Blackstone has observed, does not entertain such sublime ideas of the honour of either sex, as to lay the blame of a mutual fault on one only of the transgressors. And it is, therefore, essential to the crime of rape,

* Deuteronomy xxii. 28, 29.

rape, that the woman's will is violated by the execution. But, by a statute of Queen Elizabeth, if the crime be perpetrated on a female child under the age of *ten* years, the consent or non-consent is immaterial, as she is supposed to be of insufficient judgment. Sir Matthew Hale is even of opinion, that such profligacy committed on an infant under *twelve* years, the age of female discretion by common law, either with or without consent, amounts to a rape and felony. But the decisions of the courts have, generally, been founded on the statute above-mentioned.

A male infant, under the age of fourteen years, is deemed, by the law, incapable of committing, and therefore cannot be found guilty of a rape, from a presumed imbecility both of body and mind. This detestable crime, being executed in secrecy, and the knowledge of it being confined to the party injured, it is just that her single testimony should be adducible in proof of the fact. Yet the excellent observation of Sir Matthew Hale merits peculiar attention: "It is an accusation," says he, "easy "to be made, and harder to be proved; but "harder to be defended by the party accused, "though innocent." He then relates two extraordinary cases of malicious prosecution for this

this crime, which had fallen under his own cognizance; and concludes, "I mention these instances, that "we may be more cautious "upon trials of offences of this nature, wherein "the court and jury may, with so much ease, "be imposed upon, without great care and "vigilance; the heinousness of the offence "many times transporting the judge and jury "with so much indignation, that they are over-"hastily carried to the conviction of the person "accused thereof, by the confident testimony "of sometimes false and malicious witnesses." Collateral and concurrent circumstances of time and place;* appearances of violence on examination &c. are, therefore, necessary to be added to the mere affirmative evidence of the prosecutor. And the inspection of a surgeon is often required, to ascertain the reality of the alledged violence. On such occasions, his testimony should be given with all possible delicacy, as well as with the utmost caution. Even external signs of injury may originate from disease, of which the following examples, which have occurred in Manchester, are adduced on very respectable authorities.

A girl,

* These circumstances are particularly adverted to in the Mosaic Law. See Deut. xxii. 25, 26, 27.

A girl, about four years of age, was admitted into the Manchester Infirmary, on account of a mortification in the female organs, attended with great soreness and general depression of strength. She had been in bed with a boy, fourteen years old; and there was reason to suspect, that he had taken criminal liberties with her. The mortification increased, and the child died. The boy, therefore, was apprehended, and tried at the Lancaster assizes; but was acquitted on sufficient evidence, that several instances of a similar disease had appeared, near the same period of time, in which there was no possibility of injury or guilt. In one of these cases the body was opened after death. The disorder had been a *typhus* fever, accompanied with a mortification of the *pudenda*. There was no evident cause of this extraordinary symptom discoverable on inspection. The lumbar glands were of a dark colour; but all the *viscera* were sound. *(r)*

XVII. Concerning *nuisances*, the investigation and testimony of the faculty may be required, whenever they are of a nature offensive by the vapours which they emit; and injurious to the health of individuals, or of the community.

(r) See Notes and Illustrations, No. XVII.

nity. The law defines any thing that worketh hurt, inconvenience, or damage, to be a nuisance.* Thus if a person keep hogs, or other noisome animals, so near the house of another, that the stench incommodes him, and renders the air unwholesome, this is a nuisance; because it deprives him of the enjoyments and benefits of his habitation. A smelting house for lead, the smoke of which kills the grass and corn, and injures the cattle of a neighbouring proprietor of land, is deemed a nuisance. Dye-houses, tanning-yards &c. are nuisances, if erected so near a water-course, as to corrupt the stream. But a chandler's factory, even when situated in a crowded town, is said to be privileged from action or indictment, because candles are regarded as necessaries of life. Hawkins, however, questions the authority of this opinion, since the making of candles may be carried on in the country without annoyance.† But this is scarcely practicable in a populous neighbourhood: And as Lord Mansfield has adjudged, that, in such cases, what makes the enjoyment of being and property uncomfortable

* See Blackstone's Comment. Book III. ch. xiii.; and Book IV. ch. xiii.

† 1 Hawk. 199. Burn's Justice, vol. III. p. 239.

uncomfortable is, in the view of the law, a nuisance*; various works and trades, essential to the happiness and interest of the community, may fall under this construction. But chemistry, mechanics, and other arts and sciences, furnish methods of diminishing, or obviating almost every species of noisome vapour. And there can be no doubt that vitriol-works, aqua-fortis works, marine acid-bleaching works, the singeing of velvets &c. may be carried on with very little inconvenience to a neighbourhood, by means neither difficult nor expensive. The same observation may be applied to the business of the dyer, the fell-monger, the tanner, the butcher, and the chandler. And as these with many other disgustful trades are, in some degree, necessary in large towns, justice and policy require, that they should only be prosecuted as nuisances, when not conducted in the least offensive mode possible. To guard against arbitrary powers in municipal government, and to render the decision and investigation of such points perfectly consistent with the liberty of the subject, the reference should be made to a jury; or at least, any individual should be allowed an appeal to one, if he think himself aggrieved.

* Burron. Mansfield, 333. Burn U. S.

The frequency of fires, in large manufacturing towns, makes it expedient that magistrates, or commissioners, should be authorized to scrutinize rigidly into the causes of them, when they occur; to punish neglect or carelessness, as well as malicious intention; and to enforce suitable measures of prevention. The plans, proposed for this last very important purpose, by Mr. Hartley and Lord Stanhope, have been proved to be effectual, and are not expensive. The adoption of them, therefore, or of other means which may hereafter be discovered, should be required, under a heavy penalty, in cases deemed by insurers *doubly hazardous*.

XVIII. It is a complaint made by coroners, magistrates, and judges, that medical gentlemen are often reluctant in the performance of the offices, required from them as citizens qualified, by professional knowledge, to aid the execution of public justice. These offices, it must be confessed, are generally painful, always inconvenient, and occasion an interruption to business, of a nature not to be easily appreciated or compensated. But as they admit of no substitution, they are to be regarded as appropriate debts to the community, which neither

neither equity nor patrotism will allow to be cancelled.

When a physician or surgeon is called to give evidence, he should avoid, as much as possible, all obscure and technical terms, and the unnecessary display of medical erudition. He should deliver, also, what he advances, in the purest and most delicate language, consistent with the nature of the subject in question.—When two or more gentlemen of the faculty are to offer their opinions or testimony, it would sometimes tend to obviate contrariety, if they were to confer freely with each other, before their public examination. Intelligent and honest men, fully acquainted with their respective means of information, are much less likely to differ, than when no communication has previously taken place. Several years ago, a trial of considerable consequence occurred, relative to a large copper work; and two physicians of eminence were summoned to the assizes, to bear testimony concerning the salubrity or insalubrity of the smoke issuing from the furnaces. The evidence they offered was entirely contradictory. One grounded his testimony on the general presumption that the ores of copper contain arsenic; and consequently that the effluvia, proceeding from the roasting of them, must be poisonous because arsenical. The other had made actual experiments on the ore, employed in the works under prosecution, and on the vapours which it yielded: He was thus furnished with full proof that no arsenic was discoverable in either. But the affirmative prevailed over the negative testimony, from the authority of the physician who delivered it; an authority which he probably would not have misapplied, if he had been antecedently acquainted with the decisive trials made by his opponent. *(s)*

XIX. It is the injunction of the law, sanctioned by the solemnity of an oath, that in judicial testimony, *the truth, the whole truth,* and *nothing but the truth* shall be delivered. A witness, therefore, is under a sacred obligation to use his best endeavours that his mind be clear and collected, unawed by fear, and uninfluenced by favour or enmity. But in criminal prosecutions, which affect the life of the person accused, scruples will be apt to arise in one who, by the advantages of a liberal education, has been accustomed to serious reflection, yet has paid no particular attention to the principles of political ethics. It is incumbent, therefore,

(s) See Notes and Illustrations, No. XIX.

therefore, on gentlemen of the faculty, to settle their opinions concerning the right of the civil magistrate to inflict capital punishment; the moral and social ends of such punishment; the limits prescribed to the excrcise of the right; and the duty of a citizen to give full efficiency to the laws.

The magistrate's *right* to inflict punishment, and the ends of such punishment, though intimately connected, are in their nature distinct. The right is clearly a substitution or transfer of that which belongs to every individual, by the law of nature, viz. instant self-defence, and security from future violence or wrong. The ends are more comprehensive, extending not only to complete security against offence, but to the correction and improvement of the offender himself, and to counteract in others the disposition of offend. Penal laws are to be regulated by this standard; and the lenity or severity, with which they are executed, should, if possible, be exactly proportionate to it. In different circumstances, either personal or public considerations may preponderate: And in cases of great moral atrocity, or when the common weal is essentially injured, all regard to the reformation of a criminal is superseded; and his life is justly forfeited to the

the good of society. In the participation of the benefits of the social union, he has virtually acceded to its conditions; and the violation of its fundamental articles renders him a rebel and an enemy, to be expelled or destroyed, both for the sake of security, and as an awful warning to others. When capital punishments are viewed in this light, the most humane and scrupulous witness may consider himself as sacrificing private emotions to public justice and social order; and that he is performing an act at once beneficial to his country and to mankind. For political and moral œconomy can subsist in no community, without the steady execution of wise and salutary laws: And every atrocious act, perpetrated with impunity, operates as a terror to the innocent, a snare to the unwary, and an incentive to the flagitious. The criminal, also, who evades the sentence of justice, like one infected with the pestilence, contaminates all whom he approaches. He, therefore, who, from false tenderness or misguided conscience, has prevented conviction, by withholding the necessary proofs,* is an accessary to all

* "The oath, administered to the witness, is not only "that what he deposes shall be true, but that he shall also "depose the whole truth: *So that he is not to conceal any*

all the evils which ensue. The maxim, that *it is better ten villains should be discharged than a single person suffer by a wrong adjudication*, is one of those partial truths which are generally misapplied, because not accurately understood. It is certainly eligible that the rules and the forms of law should be so precise and immutable, as not to involve the innocent in any decision obtained by corruption, or dictated by passion and prejudice; though this should sometimes furnish an outlet for the escape of actual offenders. The plea, also, may have some validity, in crimes of a nature chiefly political (with which, however, the faculty can professionally have no concern) such as coining and forgery, or in cases wherein the punishment much exceeds the evil or turpitude of the offence. For Lord Bacon has well observed, that " over-great penalties, besides their acerbity, deaden the execution of the law."* And when they are discovered to be unjustly inflicted, its authority is impaired; its sanctity dishonoured; and veneration gives place to disgust and abhorrence.

But

" *part of what he knows, whether interrogated particularly to* " *that point or not.*" Blackstone, B. III. ch. xxiii.

* See proposal for amending the Laws of England.—Bacon's Works, 4to. vol. II. p. 542.

But the dread of *innocent blood being brought upon us*, by explicit and honest testimony, is one of those superstitions, which the nurse has taught, and which a liberal education ought to purge from the mind. And if, in the performance of our duty, innocence should unfortunately be involved in the punishment of guilt, we shall assuredly stand acquitted before God and our own consciences. The convict himself, lamentable as his fate must be regarded, may derive consolation from the reflection that, though his sentence be unjust, " he falls for " his country, whilst he suffers under the ope- " ration of those rules, by the general effect " and tendency of which the welfare of the " community is maintained and upheld."*

XX. When professional testimony is required, in cases of such peculiar malignity as to excite general horror and indignation, a virtuous mind, even though scrupulous and timid, is liable to be influenced by too violent impressions; and to transfer to the accused that dread and aversion, which, before conviction, should be confined to the crime, and as much as possible withheld from the supposed offender. If the charge, for instance, be that of parricide, accomplished

* Paley's Mor. and Polit. Phil. B. VI. ch. ix. p. 553. 4to.

accomplished by poison, and accompanied with deliberate malice, ingratitude, and cruelty; the investigation should be made with calm and unbiassed precision, and the testimony delivered with no colouring of passion, nor with any deviation from the *simplicity of truth.* When *circumstantial proofs* are adduced, they should be arranged in the most lucid order, that they may be contrasted and compared, in all their various relations, with facility and accuracy; and that their weight may be separately and collectively determined in the balance of justice. For, in such evidence, there subsists a regular gradation from the slightest presumption to complete moral certainty. And if the witness possess sufficient information in this branch of philosophical and juridical science, he will always be competent to secure himself, and, on many occasions, the court also, from fallacy and error. The Marquis de Beccaria has laid down the following excellent theorems, concerning judicial evidence: "When "the proofs of a crime are dependent on each "other, that is, when the evidence of each "witness, taken separately, proves nothing; "or when all the proofs are dependent upon "one, the number of proofs neither increases "nor diminishes the probability of the fact;

"for the force of the whole is no greater than "the force of those on which they depend; "and if this fails, they all fall to the ground. "When the proofs are independent of each "other, the probability of the fact increases in "proportion to the number of proofs; for the "falsehood of one does not diminish the vera- "city of another....... The proofs of a crime "may be divided into two classes, perfect and "imperfect. I call those perfect, which ex- "clude the possibility of innocence; imperfect, "those which do not exclude this possibility. "Of the first, one only is sufficient for con- "demnation; of the second, as many are re- "quired as form a perfect proof; that is to say, "each of these, separately taken, does not ex- "clude the possibility of innocence; it is ne- "vertheless excluded by their union."*

* Beccaria's Essay on Crimes and Punishments, chap. xiv.

AN

APPENDIX,

CONTAINING

I. *A DISCOURSE*,

ADDRESSED TO THE GENTLEMEN OF THE FACULTY;

THE OFFICERS;

THE CLERGY; AND THE TRUSTEES OF THE

INFIRMARY AT LIVERPOOL,

ON THEIR RESPECTIVE HOSPITAL DUTIES;

BY THE

REV. THOMAS BASSNETT PERCIVAL, LL. B.

Of St. John's College, Cambridge; Chaplain to the Marquis of Waterford; and to the Company of British Merchants at St. Petersburgh.

II. *NOTES AND ILLUSTRATIONS*.

- - - - LO! A GOODLY HOSPITAL ASCENDS,
IN WHICH THEY BADE EACH LENIENT AID BE NIGH,
THAT COULD THE SICK-BED SMOOTH OF THAT SAD COMPANY.
IT WAS A WORTHY EDIFYING SIGHT,
AND GIVES TO HUMAN KIND PECULIAR GRACE,
TO SEE KIND HANDS ATTENDING DAY AND NIGHT,
WITH TENDER MINISTRY, FROM PLACE TO PLACE:
SOME PROP THE HEAD; SOME, FROM THE PALLID FACE,
WIPE OFF THE FAINT COLD DEWS WEAK NATURE SHEDS;
SOME REACH THE HEALING DRAUGHT; THE WHILST TO CHACE
THE FEAR SUPREME, AROUND THEIR SOFTENED BEDS,
SOME HOLY MAN BY PRAYER ALL OPENING HEAVEN DISPREDS;

Thomson's Castle of Indolence; Canto II.

A

DISCOURSE ON HOSPITAL DUTIES,

BEING AN

ANNIVERSARY SERMON,

Preached in May 1791;

FOR THE BENEFIT OF THE INFIRMARY AT LIVERPOOL. (s)

Let us not be weary in well doing, for in due season we shall reap if we faint not. Galatians vi. 9.

IF we consider the circumstances of man, as placed in this great theatre of action; as connected with his fellow-creatures by various ties and relations; and with God himself, his creator and judge: If we consider the powers and faculties with which he is endowed, and that these are talents committed to his trust, capable of indefinite degrees of improvement, and which the Lord, at his coming, will demand with usury; we shall see the fullest reason for the apostolical injunction, *be not weary in well doing;* and rejoice in the assurance, that *in due season we shall reap, if we faint not*. The sphere of human duty has no limits to

(s) See Notes and Illustrations, No. XX.

to its extent. Every advance in knowledge widens its boundaries; every increase of power and wealth multiplies and diversifies the objects of it; and length of years evinces their unceasing succession. Therefore, *whatsoever thy hand findeth to do, do it with all thy might.* Vigour and perseverance are essential to every noble pursuit; and no virtuous effort is in vain. To be discouraged by opposition; to be alarmed by danger; or overcome by difficulty, is a state of mind unfitted for the Christian warfare.

But the present interesting occasion calls for a specific application of the precept, contained in our text. What is just and true, concerning the whole duty of man, must be equally just and true of every individual branch of moral and religious obligation. And it can require no deep research, no abstruse investigation, to work conviction on our minds, that the higher is the object we have in view, the more active and incessant should be our exertions in the attainment of it. The institution, which now claims your most serious attention, is founded on the *wisest policy;* adapted to the noblest purposes of *humanity;* and capable of being rendered subservient to the *everlasting welfare* of mankind.

The

The *wisdom* of such charitable foundations can admit of no dispute. On the lower classes of our fellow-citizens alone, we depend for food, for raiment, for the habitations in which we dwell, and for all the conveniences and comforts of life. But health is essential to their capacity for labour; and in this labour, I fear, it is too often sacrificed. An additional obligation, therefore, to afford relief, springs from so affecting a consideration. He, who at once toils and suffers for our benefit, has a multiplied claim to our support; and to withhold it would be equally chargeable with folly, ingratitude, and injustice.

But *humanity* prompts, when the still voice of wisdom is not heard. Sickness, complicated with poverty, has pleas that, to a feeling mind, are irresistible. *To weep with those that weep* was the character of our divine master; and, to the honour of our nature, we are capable of the same generous sympathy. Vain and idle, however, are the softest emotions of the mind, when they lead not to correspondent actions. And he who views the naked, without cloathing them, and those who are sick, without ministering unto them, incurs the dreadful denunciation, *Depart from me ye*

cursed

cursed into everlasting fire, prepared for the devil and his angels. For in as much as ye did it not to one of the least of these my brethren, ye did it not unto me.

It were an easy and pleasing task to enlarge on these general topics. But they come not sufficiently "home to men's business and bosoms." And honoured as I am, by being thus called to the privilege of addressing you, I feel it incumbent on me to be more appropriate, by suggesting to your candid attention, the distinct and relative duties attached to the several orders, which compose this most excellent community. Permit me, therefore, to claim your indulgence, whilst I offer, with all deference and respect, but with the plainness and freedom of gospel sincerity, a few words of exhortation:

I. To THE FACULTY;

II. To THE OFFICERS AND SUPERINTENDANTS;

III. To THE CLERGY;

And lastly, TO THE GENERAL BODY OF TRUSTEES AND CONTRIBUTORS.

I. To THE FACULTY. As man is placed by Divine Providence in a situation which involves a variety of interests and duties, often complicated

cated and mixed together, the motives which influence human actions must necessarily be mixed and complicated. Wisdom and virtue consist in the selection of those which are fit and good, and in the arrangement of all, by a just appreciation of their comparative dignity and importance. In the acceptance of your professional offices, in this Infirmary, it is presumed that you have been governed by the *love of reputation* ; by the *desire of acquiring knowledge and experience* ; and by that *spirit of philanthropy*, which delights in, and is never weary of well doing. Let us briefly consider each of these principles of action, and how they ought to be regulated.

If we analyze the *love of reputation*, as it exists in liberal and well-informed minds, it will be found to spring from the love of moral and intellectual excellence. For of what value is praise, when not founded on desert? But the consciousness of desert, by the constitution of our nature, is ever attended with self-approbation : And this delightful emotion, which is at once the concomitant and the reward of virtue, widely expands its operation, and by a social sympathy, encircles all who are the witnesses or judges of our generous deeds. From the same principle, piety itself derives its origin. For how shall he who loveth not, or is regardless of the approbation of his brother, whom he hath seen, love or regard the favour of God, whom he hath not seen!

But let us remember, not to substitute, for the legitimate and magnanimous love of fame, that spurious and sordid passion, which seeks applause by gratifying the caprices, by indulging the prejudices, and by imposing on the follies of mankind. To court the public favour by adulation, or empirical arts, is meanness and hypocrisy; to claim it, by high and assumed pretensions, is arrogance and pride; and to exalt our own character, by the depreciation of that of our competitor, is to convert honourable emulation into professional enmity and injustice.

You have been elevated by the suffrages of your fellow-citizens: You have been honoured by their favour and confidence: Rejoice in the distinction conferred upon you; fulfil with assiduity and zeal the trust reposed in you; and by being unwearied in well doing, rise to higher and higher degrees of public favour and celebrity!

The *acquisition of knowledge and experience* is a farther incentive to your generous exertions, in in this receptacle of disease and misery. It is one important design of the institution itself; which affords peculiar advantages for ascertaining the operation of remedies, and the comparative merit of different modes of medical and chirurgical treatment. For the strict rules which are enjoined; the steadiness with which their observance is enforced; and the unremitting attendance of those who are qualified to make accurate observations, and to note every symptom, whether regular or anomalous, in the diseases under cure, are circumstances incompatible with the ordinary domestic care of the sick. To avail yourselves of them, therefore, is agreeable to sound policy, and consonant to the purest justice and humanity. For every improvement in the healing art is a public good, beneficial to the poor as well as to the rich, and to the former in a proportionably greater degree, as they are more numerous, and consequently more frequently the objects of it. On this point, however, peculiar delicacy is required; and as the discretionary power, with which you are entrusted, is almost without controul, it should be exercised with the nicest honour and probity. When novelties in practice are introduced, be careful that they are conformable to reason and analogy; that no sacrifice be made to fanciful hypothesis, or experimental curiosity; that the infliction of pain or suffering be, as much as possible, avoided; and that the end in view fully warrant the means for its attainment.

But your noblest call to duty and exertion arises from the exalted *spirit of philanthropy:* And on this occasion I may address you individually, in the language of the first of orato s, to the sovereign of imperial Rome: *Nihil habet fortuna tua majus quam ut possis, nec natura melius quam ut velis, servare quam plurimos.* It is your honour and felicity to be engaged in an occupation which leads you, like our blessed Lord during his abode on earth, to go about doing good, healing the sick, and curing all manner of diseases. To you learning has opened her stores, that they may be applied to the sublimest purposes; to alleviate pain; to raise the drooping head; to renew the roses of the cheek, and the sparkling of the eye; and thus to gladden, whilst you lengthen life. Let this hospital be the theatre on which you display, with assiduous and persevering care, your science, skill, and humanity. And let the manner correspond with, and even heighten

ten the measure of your benevolence. With patience hear the tale of symptoms; silence not harshly the murmurs of a troubled mind; and by the kindness of your looks and words, evince that Christian condescension may be compatible with professional steadiness and dignity.

It is, I trust, an ill-founded opinion, that compassion is not the virtue of a surgeon. This branch of the profession has been charged with hardness of heart: And some of its members have formerly justified the stigma, by ridiculing all softness of manners; by assuming the contrary deportment; and by studiously banishing from their minds that sympathy, which they falsely supposed would be unsuitable to their character, and unfavourable to the practical exercise of their art. But different sentiments now prevail. And a distinction should ever be made between true compassion, and that unmanly pity which enfeebles the mind; which shrinks from the sight of woe; which inspires timidity; and deprives him, who is under its influence, of all capacity to give relief. Genuine compassion rouses the attention of the soul; gives energy to all its powers; suggests expedients in danger;

ger; incites to vigorous action in difficulty; and strengthens the hand to execute, with promptitude, the purposes of the head. The pity which you should repress is a turbulent emotion. The commiseration which you should cultivate is a calm principle. It is benevolence itself directed forcibly to a specific object. And the frequency of such objects diminishes not, but augments its energy: For it produces a tone or constitution of mind, constantly in unison with suffering; and prepared, on every call, to afford the full measure of relief. Appear, therefore, to your patients, to be actuated by that fellow-feeling, which nature, education, and Christianity require. Make their cases, in a reasonable degree, your own; *and whatsoever ye would that men should do unto you, do ye even so unto them.*

II. To you, the OFFICERS and SUPERINTENDANTS of this hospital, we may justly ascribe views the most pure and public-spirited. But zeal in the cause of charity, however sincere, can only be rendered usefully efficient by due attention to, and steady perseverance in the wisest means for its accomplishment. On the mistaken humanity of crowding your wards with numerous patients, by which disease is generated,

generated, and death multiplied in all its horrors; on the fatal calculations of savings in medicines, diet, or clothing; and on a strict attention to ventilation, cleanliness, and all the domestic arrangements, which have order, utility, or comfort for their objects; I trust it is needless to enlarge. But you will suffer me, I hope, to offer a few hints on the *moral* and *religious* application of the institution which you govern; a topic hitherto little noticed, though of high importance.

The visitation of sickness is a wise and kind disponsation of Providence, intended to humble, to refine, and to meliorate the heart. And its salutary influence extends beyond the sufferer, to those relatives and friends, whose office it is to minister unto him; exciting tenderness and commiseration; drawing closer the bonds of affection; and rousing to exertions, virtuous in their nature, profitable to man, and well pleasing to God. A parent, soothed and supported under the anguish of pain, by the loving kindness of his children; a husband nursed with unwearied assiduity by the partner of his bed; a child experiencing all the tenderness of paternal and maternal love, are situations which form the ground-work of domestic virtue, and domestic

domestic felicity. They leave indelible impressions on the mind, impressions which exalt the moral character, and render us better men, better citizens, and better Christians. It is wisdom, therefore, and duty, not to frustrate the benevolent constitutions of Heaven, by dissolving the salutary connections of sickness, and transporting into a public asylum those who may, with a little aid, enjoy in their own homes, benefits and consolations which, elsewhere, it is in the power of no one to confer. *(t)*

But numerous are the sufferers under sickness and poverty, to whom your hospitable doors may be opened, with the highest moral benefit to themselves and to the community. When admitted within these walls, they form one great family, of which you are the heads, and consequently responsible for all due attention to their present behaviour, and to the means of their future improvement. Withdrawn from the habitations of penury, sloth, and dirtiness; from the conversation of the loose and the profligate; and from all their associates in vice, they may here form a taste for the sweets of cleanliness; learn the power of bridling their

(t) See Notes and Illuſtrations, No. XXI.

their tongues; and be induced, by this temporary absence, to free themselves from all farther connection with their idle and debauched companions. Let it be your sedulous care to foster these excellent tendencies: Encourage in the patients every attention to neatness: Tolerate no filth or slovenliness, either in their persons or attire: Keep a strict guard on the decency of their behaviour: Urge them to active offices of kindness and compassion to each other: Furnish the convalescents with bibles, and with books of plain morality, and practical piety, suited to their capacities and circumstances; and which will neither delude the imagination, nor perplex the understanding: Oblige them to a regular attendance on the public worship of the hospital, or of their respective churches: And, agreeably to your laws, neglect not to make provision for the stated and frequent administration of the holy sacrament. There is something in this office peculiarly adapted to comfort and fortify the mind, under the pressure of poverty, pain, and sickness. In the contemplation of that love, which Christ manifested for us by his sufferings and death, all the consolation is experienced which divine sympathy can afford. *We have a high priest touched with the feeling of our infirmities,* and who holds forth to us this soothing invitation; *Come unto me all ye that are weary and heavy laden, and I will give you rest.* Promote the celebration of an ordinance, adapted thus to fill the mind with gratitude, and to alleviate every woe. And let the example of our Saviour's resignation to the appointments of God be enforced by it, who in his agony exclaimed, *Father, if it be thy will, let this cup pass from me, nevertheless not my will, but thine be done.*

III. I doubt not the cordial and entire concurrence of you, my REV. BRETHREN, the CLERGY who officiate in this hospital, in the recommendation of the holy sacrament, not only as a stated, but as a frequent ordinance of the institution. With you it will rest to obviate every objection to the rite, and to give it the full measure of spiritual efficacy. Enthusiasm and superstition cannot be dreaded in the offices of rational piety, conducted by those who are rational and pious. And you will neither betray men into false confidence, nor alarm them, when languishing under sickness and pain, with unseasonable terrors. *The*

spirit

spirit of a man will sustain his infirmity, but a wounded spirit who can bear? Under such circumstances, vain will be the aid of skill or medicine, without the supports and comforts, which it is your sacred function to afford. You can

------ "minister to a mind diseased;
" Pluck from the memory a rooted sorrow,
" Raze out the written troubles of the brain,
" And, with some sweet oblivious antidote,
" Cleanse the full bosom of that perilous stuff
" Which weighs upon the heart."

SHAKESPEARE.

Being thus the *Physicians* of the soul, you are essential constituents of this enlarged system of philanthropy. Apply, therefore, with diligence and zeal, the spiritual *medicines* which it is your office to dispense. Here you have a wide field *for exhortation, for correction, and for instruction in righteousness.* Convalescence peculiarly furmishes the *mollia tempora fandi*, the soft seasons of impressive counsel. The mind is then open to serious conviction; disposed to review past offences with contrition; and to look forward with sincere resolutions of mendment. Many diseases are the immediate consequences of vice. And he who has recently experienced

 the

the sufferings of guilt, will deeply feel its enormity; and cherish those precepts, which will secure him from relapse, and convert his past misery into future blessings.

IV. But this large aggregate of good, which it is the design of the present anniversary to commemorate, depends, for its support and extension, on the GENERAL BODY OF CONTRIBUTORS to the charity. How deeply interesting, then, are the claims, which your fellow-citizens have to make on your philanthropy! How important is it to the health of thousands, in rapid succession, that you should persevere in beneficence, and continue unwearied in well doing! Ordinary bounty terminates almost in the moment when it is bestowed. The object of it being withdrawn, solicitude and responsibility are no more. But in this noble institution, charity exerts itself in steady and unceasing operations. It is a stream ever full, yet ever flowing; and through the grace of God, I trust, will be inexhaustible. From your zeal, your concord, and liberality, these SACRED *waters of life* proceed. Be watchful that they are not poisoned in their source, nor contaminated in their progress. Let your *zeal* be be employed in searching out, and recommending proper objects of relief. *Call to you*, according to the injunction of our Saviour, *the halt, and the maimed, the lame, and the blind; for they cannot recompense you: Ye shall be recompensed at the resurrection of the just.* Suffer no prejudices, either political or religious, to contract the bounds of your charity. *Pass not by, on the other side, from a fellow-creature who has fallen amongst thieves*, because he is not of your party, of your sect, or even of your nation. But, like the good Samaritan, *have compassion on him, and let oil and wine be poured upon his wounds*, in this hospitable *Bethesda*. Guard, most sedulously guard, against the spirit of dissension. You are united in the labours of Christian love; and having one common and glorious cause, the contest should be for pre-eminence in doing good, not for the gratification of pride, the indulgence of resentment, or even for the interests of friendship. *(u)* To your liberality in contribution no appeal can be required, no new incitement can be urged. What your judgment approves; what experience has sanctioned;

(u) See Notes and Illustrations. No. XXII.

tioned; and what touches the tenderest feelings of your hearts, must have pleas that are irresistible.

It only remains, then, that we cordially unite in offering our devout supplications to the throne of grace, in behalf of all those *who are afflicted or distressed in mind, body, or estate; that it may please the God of all consolation to relieve them, according to their several necessities; giving them patience under their sufferings, and a happy issue out of all their afflictions: And finally, that we may be delivered from all hardness of heart; from all covetous desires, and inordinate love of riches; and, having been taught that all our doings, without charity, profit nothing, that this most excellent gift, the bond of peace, and of all virtues, may be poured into us abundantly, through the merits and mediation of our blessed Lord and Saviour.*

NOTES

AND

ILLUSTRATIONS.

I. *Note. Preface. Page* 1.

HOSPITAL AT MANCHESTER.

THIS institution comprehends an Infirmary, Lunatic Hospital, and Dispensary; and has now connected with it a House of Recovery, for the reception of patients ill of contagious fevers. It provides, also, for inoculation both variolous and vaccine; and for the delivery of pregnant women at their own habitations. From the 24th of June 1792, to the 24th of June 1802, the in-patients, admitted during the space of ten years, amounted to 3769; of which number 361 died: The out-patients amounted to 31,890; of which number 676 died: The home-patients amounted to 24,439; of which number 1970 died. The Lunatic Hospital was established in the year 1766; from which time to June 24 1802, the patients admitted have amounted to 1575. Of this number 627 have been cured; 212 have been relieved;

relieved; 488 have been discharged at the request of their friends; 171 have died; 8 have been deemed incurable; and 69 remained in the house on the 24th of June 1802. The House of Recovery, for the admission of patients ill of contagious fever, is appropriated to those, who, from extreme penury, are incapable of receiving proper aid in their own close and noisome habitations, or who are liable to communicate contagion to a numerous family, and, if in a crowded neighbourhood, even to perpetuate its virulence. It is attended by the physicians of the Infirmary; and is furnished with wine and medicines from the funds of that charity: But all the other expences are defrayed by an establishment, entitled the Board of Health, which commenced in the spring of 1796.

The general objects of this benevolent charity are threefold. I. To obviate the generation of diseases. II. To prevent the spread of them by contagion. III. To shorten the duration of existing diseases; and to mitigate their evils, by affording the necessary aids and comforts to those who labour under them.—I. Under the first head are comprehended—the inspection and improvement of the general accommodations of the poor;—the prohibition of such habitations,

bitations, as are so close, noisome or damp, as to be incapable of being rendered tolerably salubrious:—the removal of privies placed in improper situations:—provision for white-washing and cleansing the houses of the poor, twice every year:—attention to their ventilation, by windows with open casements, &c.: —the inspection of cotton-mills or other factories, at stated seasons; with regular returns of the condition as to health, clothing, appearance, and behaviour of the persons employed in them; of the time allowed for their refreshment, at breakfast and dinner; and of the accommodations of those who are parochial apprentices, or who are not under the immediate direction of their parents or friends: —the limitation and regulation of lodging-houses; on the establishment of *caravanseras* for passengers, or those who come to seek employment, unrecommended or unknown:—the establishment of public warm and cold baths: provision for particular attention to the cleaning of the streets, which are inhabited by the poor; and for the speedy removal of dung-hills, and every other species of filth:—the diminution, as far as is practicable, of noxious effluvia from different sources, such as those which arise from the work-houses of the fell-monger; the yards of the tanner, and the slaughter-houses of the butcher:—the superintendance of the several markets; with a view to prevent the sale of putrid flesh or fish, and of unsound flour, or other vegetable productions.

Under the second general head are included —the speedy removal of those who are attacked with symptoms of fever, from the cotton-mills, or factories, to the habitations of their parents or friends, or to commodious houses which may be set apart for the reception of the sick, in the different districts of Manchester: —the requisite attentions to preclude unnecessary communications with the sick, in the houses wherein they are confined; and to the subsequent changing and ventilation of their chambers, bedding, and apparel:—and the allowance of a sufficient time for perfect recovery, and complete purification of their clothes, before they return again to their works, or mix with their companions in labour. III. Under the third head are comprehended—medical attendance:—the care of nurses:—and supplies of medicine, wine, appropriate diet, fuel, and clothing.

From the opening of the House of Recovery on the 31st of May 1796, to the 31st of May 1802, 3210 patients have been admitted; of of whom 2939 have been cured; and 271 have died.

Note II. *Preface. Page* 2.

DISTRIBUTION OF PRINTED COPIES OF THE MEDICAL ETHICS.

When it was first recommended to me to enlarge and publish this code of professional Ethics, I felt extremely diffident in the adoption of an undertaking so liable to the charge of presumption, in an individual conscious of inadequate powers, and possessing no claim or authority to dictate rules to his medical brethren. With much solicitude, therefore, I availed myself of the aid and support of various judicious and learned friends, in different stations of life, by communicating to them printed copies of the general scheme. And I record not only with *gratitude*, but as the *necessary sanction* of my work, the names of those who have honoured it with their approbation or assistance. John Aikin, M. D.; Sir George Baker, Bart.; S. A. Bardsley, M.D.; Thomas Butterworth Bayley, esq.; Foster Bower, esq. Barrister; John Cross, esq. Barrister; James Currie, M. D.; Erasmus Darwin, M. D.; William Falconer, M. D.; John

 Ferriar,

Ferriar, M. D; Rev. Thomas Gisborne, M. A.; John Haygarth, M. D.; William Heberden, M. D.; Mr. Thomas Henry; Samuel Heywood, esq. Sergeant at law; Edward Holme, M. D.; George Lloyd, esq. Barrister; Rev. Archdeacon Paley; Sir G. O. Paul, Bart.; Robert Percival, of Dublin, M. D.; Mr. Simmons; Richard Warren, M. D.; Right Rev. Richard Watson, D. D. Bishop of Landaff; Charles White, esq.; and William Withering, M. D.

If it were not from the apprehension of swelling this long list of names, I should not omit the present opportunity of expressing my grateful acknowledgments to many other respectable friends, to whom copies of the Medical Ethics were transmitted, subsequently to the first circulation of the scheme.

Note III. *Chapt.* I. *Sect.* XVII.

SITUATION, CONSTRUCTION, AND GOVERNMENT OF HOSPITALS.

"In the town of Funchal, in the Island "of Madeira, the Infirmary in particular drew "our attention, as a model which might be "adopted in other countries with great advan-

"tage,

"tage. It consists of a long room, on one "side of which are the windows, and an altar "for the convenience of administering the sa- "crament to the sick. The other side is di- "vided into wards, each of which is just big "enough to contain a bed, and neatly lined "with gally-tiles. Behind these wards, and "parallel to the room in which they stand, "there runs a long gallery, with which each "ward communicates by a door; so that the "sick may be separately supplied with what- "ever they want, without disturbing their "neighbours." See *Voyages round the World*, published by Dr. Hawkesworth, vol. II. p. 8.

In the year 1790, I was consulted concerning the situation, structure, and government of a large county-hospital, about to be erected; and I shall here insert the hints, which I then suggested.

The SITUATION must, in some measure, be dependent on local circumstances: But, as far as is compatible with these, it should be dry, airy, moderately elevated, at a commodious distance from the town, and well supplied with salubrious water. If swampy grounds happen to be in the neighbourhood, particular attention should be paid to the winds which most frequently prevail, that it may be as little as possible

sible influenced by the vapours those winds are likely to convey. The same precaution is applicable to the smoke of the town. The hospital at Manchester is three-fourths of the year involved in smoke; by being erected on the eastern side of the town; an evil which might easily have been avoided, by the choice of an opposite site.

The STRUCTURE includes accommodation and ventilation: And the form best adapted *(mutatis mutandis)* to these essential purposes, appears to be that of the new prison at Manchester, which is constructed on the well-known plan of MR. HOWARD. The building, which forms the gate-way, will afford a large and commodious room above, for the governors of the charity; and, below, a shop for the apothecary, and a hall for the reception of out-patients, who would thus have no communication with the Infirmary; and consequently incur no risque, either of bringing or carrying back with them febrile or other contagion. The central part of the building is well adapted for kitchens, and other offices, over which the chapel might be constructed. The four *radii*, or buildings which project from the centre, might each contain six wards, fifteen feet square by thirteen high, in each story, with

with a gallery interposed. No ward should have more than two beds in it. For the contamination of the air arises chiefly from the crowding too many sick persons in one chamber: And contagion not only spreads by this means, but the patients sustain great injury from the multiplied spectacles of suffering, to which they are witnesses, in the large apartments of an hospital. Small chambers, also, have the advantage of being quickly ventilated. The three stories should be of the same height; and if the roof be lined with boards under the slates, the temperature of the highest story will be much less than usually affected by the heat of summer or cold of winter. In each gallery a room should be set apart for the convalescents, and for those patients who are able to quit their bed-chambers occasionally in the day time.

In the provision for ventilating the wards, it should be remembered, that, though adequate supplies of FRESH AIR are essential to its purity, the *temperature* of it, also, must be regarded with a view to salubrity. For cold is not only ungrateful to the feelings of the sick, commonly very acute, but in many diseases injurious by its sedative action: And it has often been suspected of giving energy to infection. The ventilation, too, should be accomplished without

out any current of wind perceptible by the patients; who, being ignorant of the nature and effects of contagion, have no apprehension of danger from it, but entertain strong prejudices against a flow of cool air; especially when in bed, or asleep. These prejudices, if they are to be deemed such, claim not only tenderness, but indulgence. For, though silenced by authority, as I have before observed, they will operate secretly and forcibly on the mind, creating fear, anxiety, and watchfulness.

The GOVERNMENT of the hospital is an object of great importance, and will demand very mature consideration. The system adopted in most of our charitable institutions, appears to me neither sufficiently comprehensive nor efficient; and some unhappy disputes in the Manchester Infirmary, induced me to draw up the following propositions, for the consideration of the trustees:

I. A committee, for the purpose of mediation, superintendance, and improvement, should be chosen, by ballot, from among the trustees: It should consist of nine gentlemen of talents, respectability, and independence, to give dignity and authority to their proceedings: It should be stiled the COUNCIL of the Infirmary; or or be distinguished by some other honourable and expressive appellation: And, when regularly convened, five members should be competent to transact business.

II. No officer of the Infirmary, nor any physician or surgeon belonging to it, should be eligible into the council.

III. No member of the council should continue in office more than three years: Three members should annually go out of office, and three others be chosen in their room: And the same gentlemen may be re-elected after the expiration of one or more years.

IV. The council should be a board of arbitration, for adjusting whatever differences or disputes may arise between the several members of the Infirmary: It should take cognizance of every thing relative to the polity of this institution, and of its appendages, the Lunatic Hospital and Dispensary: It should enquire into the progress and present state of the charity: It should suggest to the annual board of trustees, such improvements as may be deemed expedient: And it should receive, methodize, and deliberate upon the several laws or regulations, which may be proposed by the weekly board, or by any individual trustee, according to the prescribed form of notice, previous to a final decision.

V. The council should be convened fourteen days before each Quarterly Board, or oftener, if necessary: They should then communicate to the physicians and surgeons of the Infirmary, whatever laws or regulations, relative to the medical or chirurgical departments, fall under their discussion: And they should attend, either personally or by their chairman, the succeeding Quarterly or Annual Board, to state the result of their investigations, and to assist the deliberations or decisions of the general body of trustees.

VI. The physicians and surgeons of the Infirmary should be requested to form themselves into a committee, to aid the council with their experience, knowledge and advice; and to take into consideration whatever laws or regulations may be proposed, relative to their peculiar departments, before they be referred to the decision of the general body of trustees.

VII. The meetings of the committee of physicians and surgeons, should be held the day after the assembly of the council: And they should deliver, in writing, by the senior physician or surgeon, the result of their deliberations, in due time before the succeeding

Annual

Annual or Quarterly Board, to an adjourned meeting of the council.

N. B. The council may be either a permanent or a temporary institution, and subsist only during the space of two or three years, being renewable at stated periods of time, or whenever emergencies shall require such an establishment.

Note IV. *Chap.* I. *Sect.* XXVI.

HOUSE OF RECEPTION FOR PATIENTS ILL OF CONTAGIOUS FEVERS.

IN Note, No. I. it has been stated that a house of reception for patients ill of infectious fevers, now forms part of the system of the Manchester Dispensary. To aid the establishment of similar institutions in other places, I shall insert the regulations which form the polity of the House.

REGULATIONS FOR THE ADMISSION OF PATIENTS INTO THE HOUSE OF RECOVERY.

I. The physicians of the Infirmary shall be authorised to give one or two shillings, from the funds of this institution (by a ticket to the secretary of the Board of Health) to the person

 who

who shall furnish the earliest information of the appearance of Fever in any poor family, within the limits of their respective districts.

II. As soon as the secretary has received this ticket, he shall apply, or take care that application be made, to some trustee of the Board of Health, living within the district, and who is a subscriber to the Infirmary, for an immediate recommendation of the sick person as an home patient.

III. Such patients, as the physicians shall deem peculiar objects of recommendation, either on account of their extreme poverty, or of the close and crowded state of their habitations, shall be conveyed in a sedan-chair (provided with a moveable washing lining, kept for this sole purpose, and distinguished by proper marks) to the House of Recovery.

IV. The physicians shall be requested to form the necessary regulations, for the domestic government of the families of the home patients, afflicted with fever.

V. A reward, to the amount of shall be given to the heads of the family, after the cessation of the fever, on condition that they have faithfully observed the rules prescribed for cleanliness, ventilation, and the prevention of infection, amongst their neighbours. This reward

reward shall be doubled, in cases of extraordinary danger, and when the attentions have been adequate and successful.

VI. After the visitation of fever has ceased in any poor dwelling house, the sum of , or a sufficient sum, shall be allowed (to be expended under the direction of an inspector) for white-washing and cleansing the premises, and for the purchase of new bed-clothes, or apparel, in lieu of such as it may be deemed necessary to destroy, to obviate the continuance or propagation of fever.

VII. An inspector shall be appointed, in each district of the Infirmary, to aid the execution, and to enforce the observance of the foregoing regulations. And the gentlemen of the Strangers' Friend Society shall be requested to undertake this office.

INTERNAL REGULATIONS FOR THE HOUSE OF RECOVERY.

I. Every patient, on admission, shall change his infectious, for clean, linen; the face and hands are to be washed clean with lukewarm water, and the lower extremities fomented.

II. The clothes brought into the house by patients shall be properly purified and aired.

III. All

III. All linen and bed-clothes, immediately on being removed from the bodies of the patients, shall be immersed in cold water, before they are carried down stairs.

IV. All discharges from the patients shall be removed from the wards without delay.

V. The floors of the wards shall be carefully washed twice a week, and near the beds every day.

VI. Quick-lime shall be slaked in large open vessels, in every ward, and renewed whenever it ceases to bubble on the affusion of water. The walls and roofs shall be frequently washed with this mixture.

VII. No relation or acquaintance shall be permitted to visit the wards, without particular orders from one of the physicians.

VIII. No strangers shall be admitted into the wards; and the nurses shall be strictly enjoined not to receive unnecessary visits.

IX. No linen or clothes shall be removed from the House of Recovery, till they have been washed, aired, and freed from infection.

X. No convalescents shall be discharged from the house, without a consultation of the physicians.

XI. The nurses and servants of the house shall have no direct communication with the Infirmary;

Infirmary; but shall receive the medicines in the room already appropriated to messengers from the home-patients.

XII. The committee of the Strangers' Friend Society, shall be requested to undertake the office of inspecting the House of Recovery.

XIII. A weekly report of the patients admitted and discharged, shall be published in the Manchester newspapers.

XIV. When a patient dies in the wards, the body shall be removed as soon as possible, into a room appropriated to that use; it shall then be wrapt in a pitched cloth, and the friends shall be desired to proceed to the interment as early as is consistent with propriety.

XV. All provisions and attendance for the patients in this House of Recovery, shall be provided from the funds of this institution, without any communication with the Infirmary.

The establishment of fever-wards was proposed in 1774, and a few years afterward carried into complete execution by my excellent, and truly philanthropic friend Dr. Haygarth; whose life has been actively devoted to the promotion of science, the improvement of his profession, and the general good of mankind. The reader will find in his writings views

views concerning the nature, causes, and prevention of contagion, derived from philosophical principles, and confirmed by extensive and accurate observation.* These interesting subjects have lately, in a peculiar degree, engaged the attention, and employed the pens of various other distinguished writers, as appears by the works of Dr. Wall, Dr. Currie, Dr. Ferriar, and Dr. Clark.†

Note V. *Chap.* I. *Sect.* XXXI.

CAUTION OR TEMERITY IN PRACTICE.

It is the observation of an elegant writer on the subject of morals, and applicable to medical practice, that "the best character is that "which is not swayed by temper of any kind; "but alternately employs enterprise and caution, "as each is useful to the particular purpose in- "tended.

* See Haygarth's Enquiry how to prevent the Small-pox.—Sketch of a plan to exterminate the casual Small-pox.—Letter to Dr. Percival on the prevention of infectious fevers.

† See the Reports of the Society for bettering the condition and increasing the comforts of the Poor.—Dr. Stanger's Remarks on the necessity and means of suppressing contagious Fever.—Also Thoughts on the Means of preserving the Health of the Poor, by the Revd. Sir W. Clarke, Bart. and several other valuable modern works.

"tended. Such is the excellence which St· "Evremond ascribes to Mareschal TURENNE; "who displayed every campaign, as he grew "older, more temerity in his military enter- "prises; and being now, from long experi- "ence, perfectly acquainted with every inci- "dent in war, he advanced with greater firm- "ness and security, in a road so well known to "him."* Yet it is said of the great Duke of Marlborough, that ten years of such uninterrupted and splendid success as no other general could boast of, never betrayed him into a single rash action.†

That boldness in medical practice is more frequently the antecedent than the consequence of experience, is a melancholy truth; for it is generally founded either on theoretical dogmas, or on pride which disclaims authority. To the consideration of physicians, who are thus prematurely confident in their own powers, the remark of Lord Verulam may be recommended. "This is well to be weighed, that boldness "is ever blind; for it seeeth not dangers and "inconveniences; therefore it is ill in counsel, "good in execution: so that the right use of

U "bold

* Hume's Essays, vol. II. p. 284.

† See Smith's Theory of Moral Sentiments, vol. II. p. 158.

"bold persons is, that they never command in "chief, but be seconds, and under the di- "rection of others. For in counsel it is good "to see dangers, and in execution not to see "them, except they be very great."

Note VI. *Chap.* II. *Sect.* II.

TEMPERANCE OF PHYSICIANS.

"Though much has been said, and with "some truth, of the good effects of wine in "producing rapidity and vivacity of thought, "it has scarcely ever been pretended that it "favoured the exercise of discrimination and "judgment. The only persons in whom it "has ever been supposed not to have the very "opposite effects, are some gentlemen of the "faculty. The ignorant vulgar would think, "*a priori*, that, *cæteris paribus*, a physician "who was sober, would attend more accu- "rately to the case of his patient, and compare "and distinguish all circumstances better, and "judge more soundly, and prescribe more rati- "onally, than he could do when he was drunk. "But some physicians, who should be supposed "to know themselves best, and who certainly "must have known how they acquitted them- "selves in those different situations, have boasted

"that

"that they prescribed as well drunk as sober. "In this they could not be mistaken; for, whe-"ther we consider the matter physically or "logically, their boast amounts precisely to "this, that they prescribed no better when "they were sober than they did when they "were drunk; which is undoubtedly a noble "accomplishment; but it is not surely either "wonderful or rare."*

TACITUS, in his admirable treatise *De Moribus Germanorum*, has stated, that those nations—*de reconciliandis invicem inimicis, et jungendis affinitatibus, et adsciscendis principibus, de pace denique ac bello, plerumque ni conviviis consultant: tamquam nullo magis tempore aut ad simplices cogitationes pateat animus, aut ad magnas incalescat. Gens non astuta nec callida, aperit adhuc secreta pectoris licentiâ loci. Ergo detecta et nuda omnium mens posterâ die retractatur; et salva utriusque temporis ratio est. Deliberant dum fingere nesciunt: constituunt dum errare non possunt.*†

In deliberation, it may, on some peculiar occasions, be of importance to break off all

 former

* See the Introduction to Philosophical and Literary Essays, by Dr. Gregory of Edinburgh, p. 187.

† Taciti Opera à Lipsio. fol. 1627. p. 444.—The learned editor observes, in his note on this passage, *Persarum similis mos, et Cretensium, et Græcorum omnium veterum.*

former strong associations. A fit of drunkenness accomplishes this fully: Sleep has the same tendency, and hence the proverb, *I will sleep upon it*. But such deliberation bears no analogy to what is required from a physician, when he is to consider the case of a patient.

" Universal temperance," says Mr. Gis-" borne, " both in eating and drinking, is " particularly incumbent on a physician in every " period of his practice, not merely as being " essentially requisite to preserve his faculties " in that alert and unclouded state, which may " render him equally able at all times to pro-" nounce on the cases which he is called to " inspect, but because it is a virtue which he " will very frequently find himself obliged to " inculcate on his patients; and will inculcate " on them with little effect, if it be not regu-" larly exemplified in his own conduct."*

Note VII. *Chap.* II. *Sect.* III.

" A PHYSICIAN SHOULD BE THE MINISTER OF HOPE AND COMFORT TO THE SICK."

Mr. Gisborne, in one of his interesting letters to me on the subject of Medical Ethics, suggests,

* Duties of Men, vol. II. p. 139. Note.

suggests, that it would be adviseable to add, *as far as truth and sincerity will admit.* " I " know very well," says he, " that the sen- " tence, as it now stands, conveys to you, and " was meant by you to convey to others, the " same sentiment which it would express after " the proposed addition. But if I am not mis- " taken in my idea, that there are few profes- " sional temptations to which medical men are " more liable, and frequently from the very " best principles, than that of unintentionally " using language to the patient and his friends, " more encouraging than sincerity would vin- " dicate, on cool reflection; it may be right " scrupulously to guard the avenues against such " an error."

In the *Enquiry into the Duties of Men*, the same excellent moralist thus delivers his sentiments more at large. " A professional " writer, speaking, in a work already quoted,* " respecting the performance of surgical opera- " tions in hospitals, remarks, that it may be a " salutary, as well as an humane act, in the at- " tending physician, occasionally to assure the " patient that every thing goes on well, *if that* " *declaration can be made with truth.* This " restriction,

* Percival's Medical Ethics. Chap. I.

"restriction, so properly applied to the case in "question, may with equal propriety be ex-"tended universally to the conduct of a phy-"sician, when superintending operations per-"formed, not by the hand of a surgeon, but "by nature and medicine. Humanity, we "admit, and the welfare of the sick man "commonly require, that his drooping spirits "should be revived by every encouragement "and hope, which can honestly be suggested "to him. But truth and conscience forbid the "physician to cheer him by giving promises, "or raising expectations, which are known, "or intended to be, delusive. The physician "may not be bound, unless expressly called "upon, invariably to divulge, at any specific "time, his opinion concerning the uncertainty "or danger of the case: but he is invariably "bound never to represent the uncertainty or "danger as less than he actually believes it to "be; and whenever he conveys, directly or "indirectly, to the patient or to his family, any "impression to that effect, though he may be "misled by mistaken tenderness, he is guilty "of positive falsehood. He is at liberty to say "little; but let that little be true. St. Paul's "direction,

"direction, *not to do evil, that good may come,* "is clear, positive, and universal."*

Whether this subject be viewed as regarding general morality, or professional duty, it is of high importance; and we may justly presume, that it involves considerable difficulty and intricacy, because opposite opinions have been advanced upon it by very distinguished writers. The ANCIENTS, though sublime in the abstract representations of virtue, are seldom precise and definite in the detail of rules for its observance. Yet in some instances they extend their precepts to particular cases: And Cicero, in the Third Book of his Offices, expressly admits of limitations to the absolute and immutable obligation of fidelity and truth.

The maxim of the poet, also, may be adduced as intended to be comprehensive of the moral laws, by which human conduct is to be governed:

> —— Sunt certi denique fines,
> Quos ultrá citráque nequit consistere réctum.†

The early FATHERS of the Christian church, Origen, Clement, Tertullian, Lactantius, Chrysostom, and various others, till the period of St.

* Duties of Men, vol. II. p. 148.

† Horat. Sat. Lib. I. Sat. I. 106.

St. Augustine, were latitudinarians on this point. But the holy father last mentioned, if I mistake not, in the warmth of his zeal, declared that he would not utter a lie, though he were assured of gaining Heaven by it. In this declaration there is a fallacy, by which Augustine probably imposed upon himself. For a lie is always understood to consist in a *criminal* breach of truth, and therefore under no circumstances can be justified. It is alledged, however, that falsehood may lose the essence of lying, and become even praise-worthy, when the adherence to truth is incompatible with the practice of some other virtue of still higher obligation. This opinion almost the whole body of CIVILIANS adopt, with full confidence of its rectitude. The sentiments of Grotius may be seen at large in the satisfactory detail which he has given of the controversy relating to it.*

Puffendorff, who may be regarded as next to this great man in succession as well as authority, delivers the following observations in his *Law of Nature and Nations*, which are pointedly

* See the second, third, and fourth paragraphs of the 10th Sect. Cap. I. Lib. III. of Grotius de Jure Bell. ac Pac.—Also the 14th, 15th, and 16 Sections of the same Chapter.

edly applicable to the present subjects, yet carried assuredly to a very reprehensible extent: "Since those we talk to may often be in such "circumstances, that if we should tell them the "downright truth of the matter, it would pre-"judice them, and would incapacitate us for pro-"curing that lawful end we propose to ourselves "for their good; we may in these cases use a "fictitious or figurative way of speech, which "shall not directly represent to our hearers our "real thoughts and intentions: For when a "man is desirous, and it is his duty, to do a "piece of service, he is not bound to take "measures that will certainly render his at-"tempts unsuccessful."*—"Those are by no "means guilty of lying, who, for the better "information of children, or other persons not "capable of relishing the naked truth, enter-"tain them with fictions and stories: Nor those "who invent something that is false, for the "sake of a good end, which by the plain "truth, they could not have compassed; as, "suppose, for protecting an innocent, for ap-"peasing a man in his passion, for *comforting* "*the afflicted*, for *animating the timorous*, for "*persuading a nauseating patient to take his* "*physic*, for overcoming an obstinate humour, "for making an ill design miscarry."†

* Spavan's Puffendorff, vol. II. Chap. I. p. 6. † Ibid. p. 9.

Several modern ETHICAL WRITERS, of considerable celebrity, have been no less explicit and indulgent on this question. Amongst these, it may suffice to cite the testimony of the late Dr. Francis Hutcheson of Glasgow; of whom it is said by his excellent biographer, that "he abhorred the least appearance of deceit either in word or action."* "When in "certain affairs," says he, "it is known that "men do not conceive it an injury to be deceived, there is no crime in false speech "about such matters.—No man censures a "physician for deceiving a patient too much "dejected, by expressing good hopes of him; "or by denying that he gives him a proper "medicine which he is foolishly prejudiced "against: the patient afterwards will not reproach him for it.—Wise men allow this liberty to the physician in whose skill and "fidelity they trust: Or if they do not, there "may be a just plea from necessity."†—"These "pleas of necessity some would exclude by a "maxim of late received, *We must not do evil* "*that good may come of it.* The author of "this

* Dr. Leechman's Biographical Preface to Hutcheson's System of Moral Philosophy, p. 26.

† Hutcheson's System of Moral Philosophy, vol. I. p. 32, 33.

" this maxim is not well known. It seems by " a passage in St. Paul, that Christians were " reviled as teaching that since the mercy " and veracity of God were displayed by the " obstinate wickedness of the Jews, they " should continue in sin, that this good might " ensue from it. He rejects the imputation " upon his doctrine; and hence some take up " the contradictory proposition as a general " maxim of great importance in morality. " Perhaps it has been a maxim among St. " Paul's enemies, as they upbraid him with " counteracting it. Be the author who they " please, it is of no use in morals, as it is quite " vague and undetermined. Must one do no- " thing for a good purpose, which would have " been evil without this reference? It is evil " to hazard life without a view to some good; " but when it is necessary for a public interest, " it is very lovely and honourable. It is cri- " minal to expose a good man to danger for " nothing; but it is just even to force him into " the greatest dangers for his country. It is " criminal to occasion any pains to innocent " persons, without a view to some good: but " for restoring of health we reward chirur- " geons for scarifyings, burnings, and amputa- " tions. *But*, say they, *such actions, done for* "*these ends, are not evil. The maxim only* "*determines that we must not do, for a good* "*end, such actions as are evil even when done* "*for a good end.* But this proposition is iden-"tic and useless; for who will tell us next, "what these actions, sometimes evil, are, "which may be done for a good end? and "what actions are so evil that they must not "be done even for a good end? The maxim "will not answer this question; and truly it "amounts only to this trifle; *you ought not* "*for any good end to do what is evil, or what* "*you ought not to do even for a good end.*"*

Dr. Johnson, who admits of some exception to the Law of Truth, strenuously denies the right of telling a lie to a sick man for fear of alarming him. "You have no business with "consequences," says he, "you are to tell the "truth. Besides, you are not sure what effect "your telling him that he is in danger may "have. It may bring his distemper to a crisis, "and that may cure him. Of all lying I have "the greatest abhorrence of this, because I "believe it has been frequently practised on "myself."†

If

* Hutcheson's System of Mor. Phil. vol. II. p. 132.

† See Boswell's Life of Johnson, p. 570.

If the medical reader wishes to investigate this nice and important subject of casuistry, he may consult *Grotius de Jure Bell. ac Pacis;* Puffendorff; Grove's Ethics; Balguy's Law of Truth; Cambray's Telemachus; Butler; Hutcheson; Paley; and Gisborne. Every practitioner must find himself occasionally in circumstances of very delicate embarrassment, with respect to the contending obligations of veracity and professional duty: And when such trials occur, it will behove him to act on fixed principles of rectitude, derived from previous information, and serious reflection. Perhaps the following brief considerations, by which I have conscientiously endeavoured to govern my own conduct, may afford some aid to his decision.

Moral truth, in a professional view, has two references; one to the party to whom it is delivered, and another to the individual by whom it is uttered. In the first, it is a *relative duty*, constituting a branch of justice; and may be properly regulated by the divine rule of equity prescribed by our Saviour, to *do unto others, as we would*, all circumstances duly weighed, *they should do unto us*. In the second, it is a *personal duty*, regarding solely the sincerity, the purity, and the probity of the physician himself.

himself. To a patient, therefore, perhaps the father of a numerous family, or one whose life is of the highest importance to the community, who makes enquiries which, if faithfully answered, might prove fatal to him, it would be a gross and unfeeling wrong to reveal the truth. His right to it is suspended, and even annihilated; because its beneficial nature being reversed, it would be deeply injurious to himself, to his family, and to the public: And he has the strongest claim, from the trust reposed in his physician, as well as from the common principles of humanity, to be guarded against whatever would be detrimental to him. In such a situation, therefore, the only point at issue is, whether the practitioner shall sacrifice that delicate sense of veracity, which is so ornamental to, and indeed forms a characteristic excellence of the virtuous man, to this claim of professional justice and social duty. Under such a painful conflict of obligations, a wise and good man must be governed by those which are the most imperious; and will therefore generously relinquish every consideration, referable only to himself. Let him be careful, however, not to do this, but in cases of real emergency, which happily seldom occur; and to guard his mind sedulously against the injury it may sustain

tain by such violations of the native love of truth.

I shall conclude this long note with the two following very interesting biographical facts. The husband of the celebrated Arria, Cæcinna Pætus, was very dangerously ill. Her son was also sick at the same time, and died. He was a youth of uncommon accomplishments; and fondly beloved by his parents. Arria prepared and conducted his funeral in such a manner, that her husband remained entirely ignorant of the mournful event which occasioned that solemnity. Pætus often enquired with anxiety, about his son; to whom she chearfully replied, that he had slept well, and was better. But if her tears, too long restrained, were bursting forth, she instantly retired, to give vent to her grief; and when again composed, returned to Pætus with dry eyes, and a placid countenance, quitting, as it were, all the tender feelings of the mother, at the threshold of her husband's chamber.*

Lady Russel's only son, Wriothesley, Duke of Bedford, died of the small-pox in May 1711, in the 31st year of his age. To this affliction succeeded, in Nov. 1711, the loss of her daughter,

* Plin. Epist. 16. Lib. III.

ter, the Duchess of Rutland, who died in child-bed. Lady Russell, after seeing her in the coffin, went to her other daughter, married to the Duke of Devonshire, from whom it was necessary to conceal her grief, she being at that time in child-bed likewise; therefore she assumed a chearful air, and with astonishing resolution agreeable to truth, answered her anxious daughter's enquiries with these words: "I have seen your sister out of bed to-day."*

Note VIII. *Chap.* II. *Sect.* V.

THE PRACTICE OF A PRIOR PHYSICIAN SHOULD BE TREATED WITH CANDOUR, AND JUSTIFIED SO FAR AS TRUTH AND PROBITY WILL PERMIT.

Montaigne, in one of his essays, treats, with great humour, of physic and physicians; and makes it a charge against them, that they perpetually direct variations in each others prescriptions. "Whoever saw," says he, "one physician approve of the prescription of another, without taking something away, or adding something to it? By which they sufficiently

* Note to the Letters of Lady Russel, 4to. Letter 149, p. 204.

ently betray their act, and make it manifest to us, that they therein more consider their own reputation, and consequently their profit, than their patient's interest."*

Note IX. *Chap.* II. *Sect.* IX.

THEORETICAL DISCUSSIONS SHOULD BE GENERALLY AVOIDED.

THIS rule is not only applicable to consultations, but to any reasonings on the nature of the case, and of the remedies prescribed, either with the patient himself or his friends. It is said by my lamented friend Mr. Seward, in his entertaining anecdotes, that the late Lord Mansfield gave this advice to a military gentleman, who was appointed governor of one of our islands in the West-Indies, and who expressed his apprehensions of not being able to discharge his duty as chancellor of his province. "When you decide, never give reasons for your decision. You will in general decide well; yet may give very bad reasons for your judgment."†

Y *Note*

* *Montaigne's Essays*, Book II. Ch. XXXVII. p. 703.—Consult also the same Chapter, page 719.

† Anecdotes of distinguished persons, Vol. II. p. 361.

Note X. *Chap.* II. *Sect.* XI.

REGULAR ACADEMICAL EDUCATION.

"It has been the general opinion," says Dr. Johnson, "that Sydenham was made a physician by accident and necessity; and Sir R. Blackmore reports, in the preface to his Treatise on the Small-pox, that he engaged in practice without any preparatory study, or previous knowledge of the medicinal sciences; affirming, that when he was consulted by him what books he should read to qualify him for the said profession, he recommended Don Quixote. That he recommended Don Quixote to Blackmore (continues Dr. Johnson) we are not allowed to doubt; but the relator is hindered, by the self-love which dazzles all mankind, from discovering, that he might intend a satire, very different from a general censure of all the ancient and modern writers on medicine; since he might perhaps mean, either seriously, or in jest, to insinuate, that Blackmore was not adapted by nature to the study of physic; and that, whether he should read Cervantes or Hippocrates, he would be equally unqualified for practice, and equally unsuccessful in it. Whatsoever was his meaning, nothing is more evident than

than that it was a transient sally of an imagination warmed with gaiety; or the negligent effusion of a mind intent upon some other employment, and in haste to dismiss a troublesome intruder." Sydenham himself has declared, that after he determined upon the profession of physic, he applied in earnest to it, and spent several years in the University of Oxford, before he began to practise in London. He travelled afterwards to Montpellier in quest of more information; so far was he from any con tempt of academical institutions; and so far from thinking it reasonable to learn physic by experiments alone, which must necessarily be made at the hazard of life."*

But it is highly injurious to the usefulness and honour of the profession, to suppose the education of a physician may be confined to the pursuit of medicine as an *art*. Sir W. Blackstone, in his Introduction to his Commentaries on the Laws of England, has reprobated the custom of placing the juridical student at the desk of some skilful attorney, in order to initiate him early in all the depths of practice, and to render him more dexterous in the mechanical part of business. This illiberal path to the bar

* See Johnson's Life of Sydenham.

is not to be sanctioned, he observes, by a few particular instances of persons, who, through the force of transcendant genius, have been able to overcome every disadvantage. And he points out, in very forcible terms, and with sound argument, how essential it is to the lawyer to form his sentiments by the perusal of the purest classical authors; to learn to reason with precision, by the simple but clear rules of unsophisticated logic; to fix the attention, and steadily to pursue truth through the most intricate deductions, by an acquaintance with mathematical demonstration; and to acquire enlarged conceptions of nature and of art, by a view of the several branches of experimental philosophy. Now if this be the *vantage ground*, to adopt the language of Lord Bacon, from which the study of the law should commence, it ought to be deemed at least equally necessary to qualify for the prosecution of medicine—a science which has man, as a compound of matter and mind, for its subject, and an infinitude of substances derived from the animal, vegetable, and mineral kingdoms for its instruments. This sentiment seems to have been early prevalent in the celebrated school of physic, established at Salerno in Italy. For it was enacted, A. D. 1237, by the heads of colleges there, that the pupils

pupils should be bound to pass three years in the acquisition of philosophy, and five subsequent years in that of medicine.* The like regulations were afterwards adopted in other Universities; but in various countries have fallen into disuse.

On the first revival of learning in Europe, science was held in the highest estimation; and the three faculties of law, physic, and divinity assumed

* Vide Bulæi Hist. Univers. Paris, vol. p. 158.—Henry's History of Great Britain, Vol. VIII. p. 206.

Dr. Freind, in his *Hist. Medicinæ*, has given a somewhat different account of the celebrated School of Salernum. "*Sunt in eo decem Doctores, qui sibi invicem, juxta "creationis ordinem, succedunt. Candidatorum examinatio "severissima est, que fit aut in Guleni Therapeuticis, aut in "primo primi Canonis Avicennæ, aut in Aphorismis. Is qui "Doctoratum ambit unum ac viginti annos habere debet (verum "hic lapsum subesse autumo, cum scribendum sit viginti quin-"que vel septem) ac testimonia proferre, quæ per septem annos "eum Medicinæ studuisse doceant. Quod si inter Chirurgos "recipi cupiat, Anatomiam per anni Spatium didicisse hunc "oportet: jurandum ei est, fidelem se ac morigerum Societati "futurum, præmia a pauperibus oblata recusaturum, neque "Pharmacopolarum lucri participem fore. Tum liber in "ejus manum traditur, annulus digito induitur, Caput laurea "redimitur, atque ipse osculo dimittitur. Multá alia Statuta "sunt ad Praxeos ordinationem pertinentia; Pharmacopolæ "præsertim, ut juxta Medici præcepta componant Medica-"menta, et ut ea certo pretio divendant, obligantur.*

I. Freind Opera Med. Pag. 537.

sumed particular honours and privileges. Academical degrees were conferred on their members; and these titles, with the rank annexed to them, were admitted *ubique gentium;* being, like the order of knighthood, of universal validity. Doctors indeed contended sometimes with knights for precedence, and the disputes were not unfrequently terminated by advancing the former to the dignity of knighthood. It was even asserted that a doctor had a right to that title, without creation.*

Note XI. *Chap.* II. *Sect.* XVI.

PECUNIARY ACKNOWLEDGMENTS.

THE following fact, related in Dr. Johnson's Life of Addison, is applicable to the professional conduct of physicians towards their friends. "When Addison was in office (under the Duke of Wharton, as Lord Lieutenant of Ireland) he made a law to himself, as Swift has stated, never to remit his regular fees in civility to his friends.

* Consult *Seb. Bachmeisteri Antiquitàtes Rostoch*; *Crevier Hist. de l'Univers. de Paris*; and Dr. Robertson's Proofs and Illustrations, annexed to his View of the State of Europe.—Hist. Charles V. vol. I. p. 387, 8vo.

friends. "For," said he, "I may have an hundred friends, and if my fee be two guineas, I shall, by relinquishing my right, lose two hundred guineas, and no friend gain more than two; there is therefore no proportion between the good imparted, and the evil suffered."* In recording Mr. Addison's *prudential* conduct, his probity, with respect to pecuniary acknowledgments, should not be unnoticed. In a letter, relative to the case of Major Dunbar, he says, "And now, Sir, believe me, when I assure you, I never did, nor ever will, on any pretence whatsoever, take more than the stated or customary fees of my office. I might keep the contrary practice concealed from the world, were I capable of it; but I could not from myself; and I hope I shall always fear the reproaches of my own heart, more than those of all mankind."†

At a period when empirics and empiricism seem to have prevailed much in Rome, the exorbitant demands of medical practitioners, particularly for certain secret compositions which they dispensed, induced the Emperor Valentinian to ordain, that no individual of the faculty should

* See Johnson's Lives of the Poets.

† Idem.

should make an express charge for his attendance on a patient; nor even avail himself of any promise of remuneration during the period of sickness; but that he should rest satisfied with the donative voluntarily offered at the close of his ministration.* By the same law, however, the Emperor provided that one practitioner, at least, should be appointed for each of the fourteen sections into which the Roman metropolis was divided, with special privileges, and a competent salary for his services; thus indirectly, yet explicitly acknowledging that a physician has a full claim in equity to his professional emoluments. Is it not reasonable, therefore, to conclude, that what subsisted as a *moral right*, ought to have been demandable, under proper regulations, as a *legal right?* For it seems to be the office of law to recognize and enforce that which natural justice recognizes and sanctions.

The Roman advocates were subject to the like restrictions, and from a similar cause. For their rapacity occasioned the revival of the Cincian ordinance—"*quâ cavetur antiquitùs, ne quis ob causam orandam pecuniam donumve accipiat.*" But Tacitus relates, that when

* *Vide Cod. Theodos. Lib. XIII. Tit. III.*

when the subject was brought into discussion before Claudius Cæsar, amongst other arguments in favour of receiving fees, it was forcibly urged, *sublatis studiorum pretiis, etiam studia peritura;* and that, in consequence, the prince "*capiendis pecuniis posuit modum, usque ad dena sestertia, quæ egressi repetundarum tenerentur.**

A precise and invariable *modus*, however, would be injurious both to the barrister and the physician, because the fees of each ought to be measured by the value of his time, the eminence of his character, and by his general rule of practice. This rule, with its antecedents, being well known, a *tacit compact* is established, restrictive on the claims of the practitioner, and binding on the probity of the patient. Law cannot properly, by its ordinances, establish the custom, which will and ought to vary in different situations, and under different circumstances. But a court of judicature, when formally appealed to, seems to be competent to authorize it if just, and to correct it if unjust. Such decisions could not wholly change the honorary nature of fees; because they would continue to be increased, at the discretion of the affluent, according to

 their

* Annal. Lib. XI. Pag. 168. Edit. Lipsii.

their liberality and grateful sense of kind attentions; and diminished, at the option of the physician, to those who may, from particular circumstances, require his beneficence.

From the Roman code, the established usage, in different countries of Europe, relative to medical fees, has probably originated. This usage, which constitutes common law, seems to require considerable modification to adapt it to the present state of the profession. For the general body of the faculty, especially in the united kingdoms of Great-Britain and Ireland, are held in very high estimation, on account of their liberality, learning, and integrity: * And it would be difficult to assign a satisfactory

* Of this truth, it has been my duty and inclination to offer several proofs, of unquestionable authority, in different parts of the present work. Two additional ones now occur to my recollection, which I shall here insert. Mr. Pope, writing to Mr. Allen concerning his obligations to Dr. Mead and other physicians, about a month before his death, says, "There is no end of my kind "treatment from the faculty. They are in general the "most amiable companions and the best friends, as well "as the most learned men I know."—The Rev. Dr. Samuel Parr, in a letter, with which he honoured me in September 1794, thus expresses himself: "I have long "been in the habit of reading on medical subjects; and "the great advantage I have derived from this circum- "stance

a satisfactory reason why they should be excluded from judicial protection, when the just remuneration of their services is wrongfully with-held. Indeed a medical practitioner, one especially who is settled in a provincial town, or in the country, may have accumulated claims from long-protracted and often expensive attendance; and his pecuniary acknowledgments may be refused from prejudice, from captiousness, from parsimony, or from dishonesty. Under such circumstances considerations of benevolence, humanity, and gratitude, are wholly set aside: For when disputes arise, they must be suspended or extinguished; and the question at issue, can alone be decided on the principles of *commutative justice*.

Note XII. *Chap.* II. *Sect.* XXX.

PUBLIC WORSHIP, SCEPTICISM, AND INFIDELITY.

The neglect of social worship, with which physicians have been too justly charged, may be traced, in many instances, to the period of their

" stance is, that I have found opportunities for conver- " sation and friendship with a class of men, whom after " a long and attentive survey of literary characters, I " hold to be the most enlightened professional persons in " the whole circle of human arts and sciences."

their academical education, particularly in the universities where young men are permitted to live at large, and are subject to no collegiate discipline. Sunday, affording a recess from public lectures, is devoted, by those who are ardent in study, to a review of the labours of the past week; to preparations for medical or scientific discussions in the societies of which they are members; or to other pursuits, belonging to their profession, but unconnected with religion. The idle and the gay, in such situations, are eager to avail themselves of opportunities so favourable to their taste for recreation, or to their aversion to business and confinement. In each of these classes, though actuated by different principles, there is much danger that devotional impressions will be gradually impaired, for want of stated exercise and renewal: And a foundation will thus be laid for habitual and permanent indifference, in future life, to divine services, whenever medical avocations furnish a *salvo* to the mind, and a plausible excuse to the world, for non-attendance on them. This coldness of heart, this moral insensibility, should be sedulously counteracted before it has acquired an invincible ascendancy. No apology should be admitted for absence from the stated offices of piety,

piety, but that of duties to be performed of immediate and pressing necessity. When the church is entered with just views, it will be found that there is a sympathy in religious homage, which at once inspires and heightens devotion: And that to hold communion with God in concert with our families, our friends, our neighbours, and our fellow-citizens, is the highest privilege of human nature. But with a full conviction of the obligation of public worship, as a social institution founded on common consent, and enjoined by legal authority; as a moral duty connecting us by the most endearing ties with our brethren of mankind, who are joint dependants with ourselves, on the pardon, the protection, and the bounty of God; and as a debt of general homage to our creator, benefactor, and judge; yet there may subsist in a devout and benevolent mind scruples, respecting doctrines and forms, sufficient to produce an alienation from the sacred offices of the temple. Such doubts, when they originate from serious enquiry, and are not the result of fastidiousness or arrogance, have a claim to tenderness and indulgence; because, to act in contradiction to them, whilst they subsist, would be a vioation of sincerity, amounting in some cases

to

to the guilt of hypocrisy. But in a country where private judgment is happily under no restraint, and where so great a diversity of sects prevail, it will be strange, if a candid and well-informed man can find no christian denomination, with which he might accord in spirit and in truth. Sir Thomas Brown, in the statement which he has given in his *Religio Medici*, seems to have allowed himself on these points very extensive latitude.—" We have reformed " from them, viz. the Papists, not against " them—and therefore I am not scrupulous " to converse and live with them, to enter " their churches in defect of ours, and either " pray with them or for them. I could never " perceive that a resolved conscience may not " adore her creator any where, especially in " places devoted to his service; where if their " devotions offend him, mine may please him; " if theirs profane it, mine may hallow it. I " could never hear the *Ave Maria* bell with" out an elevation, or think it a sufficient " warrant, because they erred in one circum" stance, for me to err in all—that is in silence " and dumb contempt: Whilst therefore they " direct their devotions to the virgin, I offer " mine to God, and rectify the errors of their " prayers by rightly ordering my own."

But

But authority, much more respectable than that of Sir Thomas Brown, may be adduced in favour of the spirit of catholicism in christian communion. Mr. Locke, a short time before his death, received the sacrament according to the rites of the church of England, though it is evident from his writings that he dissented from many of her doctrines. When the office was finished, he told the minister—" that he was in perfect charity with all men, and in sincere communion with the church of Christ, by what name soever it might be distinguished.*—Dr. David Hartley was originally intended for the clerical profession, but was prevented from going into holy orders by his scruples concerning subscription to the thirty-nine articles. He continued, however, to the end of his life, a well-affected member of the establishment, approving of its practical doctrines, and conforming to its public worship." He was a catholic christian, says his son and biographer, in the most extensive and literal sense of the term. On the subject of religious controversy, he has left the following testimony of his sentiments:—" The great " differences of opinion and contentions, which " happen

* See Brit. Biog. vol. VII. page 13.

"happen on religious matters, are plainly ow-"ing to the violence of men's passions more "than to any other cause. When religion has "had its due effect in restraining these, and "begetting true candour, we may expect a "unity of opinion both in religious and other "matters, as far as is necessary for useful and "practicable purposes."

These examples of the conduct of wise and conscientious christians evince that, in their estimation, forms, ceremonies, and doctrines, are of a moment subordinate to the benefits and obligations of social worship. But they are not adduced to sanction an *indifference*, either to religious rites, or religious truth. The mind will always be in the best frame for holy exercises, when the modes by which they are conducted, are consonant to its sentiments of propriety and rectitude. And that church should be habitually resorted to, if practicable, the public services of which accord most satisfactorily with the views of the individual, concerning the attributes of God, and the revelation of his will and promises to man. No personal friendship, no party connection, no professional interest should be allowed to predominate in the choice. For genuine piety, which is the joint offspring of reason and of sentiment,

sentiment, admits of no substitutions. It consists in a full conviction of the understanding, accompanied with correspondent affections of the heart; and in its exercises calls forth their united and noblest energies.

It will not be foreign to the subject of this note to investigate briefly, the imputation of scepticism and infidelity, which has been laid against the medical faculty. The Rev. Dr. Samuel Parr, whose candour is unquestionable, and whose learning and genius entitle him to the highest respect, has lately sanctioned it, as will appear by the following passage from his *Remarks on the Statement of Dr. Charles Combe*, pages 82, 83.—" While I allow," says he, " that peculiar and important advantages arise from the appropriate studies of the three liberal professions, I must confess, that in erudition, in science, and in habits of deep and comprehensive thinking, the pre-eminence, in some degree, must be assigned to physicians. The propensity which some of them have shewn to scepticism, upon religious topics, is indeed to be seriously lamented; and it may be satisfactorily explained, I think, upon metaphysical principles, which evince the strength rather than the weakness of the human mind, when contemplating, under certain circumstances, the multiplicity and energy of physical causes. But I often console myself with reflecting on the sounder opinions of Sir Thomas Browne, Sydenham, Boerhaave, and Hartley, in the days that are past; and of our own times, posterity will remember that they were adorned by the virtues, as well as the talents of a Gregory, a Heberden, a Falconer, &c."

Mr. Gisborne, in his *Enquiry into the Duties of Men, in the higher and middle Classes of Society*, a work to which I have already referred, as an admirable system of practical and appropriate ethics, has very explicitly and forcibly delivered his sentiments on this interesting subject. "The charge," he says, "may have been made on partial and insufficient grounds; but the existence of it should excite the efforts of every conscientious physician, to rescue himself from the general stigma. It should stimulate him, not to affect a sense of religion which he does not entertain, but openly to avow that which he actually feels. If the charge be in some measure true, it is of importance, to the physician, to ascertain the causes from which the fact has originated, that he may be the more on his guard against their influence. The following circumstances may not have been without their weight. They who

who are accustomed to deep researches into any branch of philosophical science; and find themselves able to explain, to their own satisfaction, almost every phænomenon, and to account, as they apprehend, for almost every effect, by what are termed natural causes, are apt to acquire extravagant ideas of the sufficiency of human reason on all subjects: and thus learning to doubt the necessity, become prejudiced against the belief of divine revelation. In the next place, they who justly disclaim the empire of authority in medical theories, may carelessly proceed to regard religious doctrines as theories, resting on no other foundation, and deserving of no better fate. Thirdly, it is to be observed, that men may be divided into two distinct classes, with respect to the sort of testimony on which they receive truths of any kind. They who are chiefly addicted to investigations and reasonings, founded on analogy, look primarily and with extreme partiality to that species of evidence; and if the thing asserted appear contrary to the common course of nature, more especially if it militate against any theory of their own (and such persons are much disposed to theorize) they are above measure reluctant to admit the reality of it; and withhold their assent until such a number of particular proofs, incapable of of being resolved into fraud or misconception, is produced, as would have been far more than sufficient to convince an unbiassed judgment. Whereas other men, little used to analogical enquiries, look not around for such testimony, either in support or in refutation of an extraordinary circumstance affirmed to them; but readily give credit to the fact on its own distinct proofs, or from confidence in the veracity and discernment of the relator. It is evident that physicians are to be ranked in the class first described, and are consequently liable to its prejudices. And it is equally evident, that those prejudices will render all, on whom they fasten, particularly averse to recognize the truth of miracles; and will probably prevent them from examining, with impartiality, the evidence of a religion founded on miracles, and perhaps from examining it at all. Fourthly; to the preceding circumstances must be added the neglect of divine wc.ship, too customary among persons of the medical profession. This neglect seems to have contributed not only to excite and strengthen the opinion of their scepticism and infidelity; but sometimes to produce scepticism and infidelity itself. For it is a natural progress, that he who habitually disregards the public duties of religion, should soon

soon omit those which are private; should speedily begin to wish that religion may not be true; should then proceed to doubt its truth; and at length should disbelieve it." Vol. II. p. 192, edit. 4.

The late Dr. Gregory, of Edinburgh, anxious to support the honour of a profession which he loved, and of which he was a distinguished ornament, very strenuously repels the charge, against it, of scepticism and infidelity. Though his excellent lectures are, doubtless, in the hands of most physicians, yet I am tempted to make a transcript from them, because I wish the present important subject to be viewed in the several lights, in which it has been presented to the mind by different writers, of acknowledged probity, information, and judgment. "I think the charge," he observes, "ill founded, and will venture to say, that the most eminent of our faculty have been distinguished for real piety. I shall only mention as examples, Harvey, Sydenham, Arbuthnot, Boerhaave, Stahl, and Hoffman.—It is easy, however, to see whence this calumny has arisen. Men whose minds have been enlarged by knowledge, who have been accustomed to think, and to reason upon all subjects with a generous freedom, are not apt to become bigots

bigots to any particular sect or system. They can be steady to their own principles, without thinking ill of those who differ from them; but they are impatient of the authority and controul of men, who would lord it over their consciences, and dictate to them what they are to believe. This freedom of spirit, this moderation and charity for those of different sentiments, have frequently been ascribed, by narrow-minded people, to secret infidelity, scepticism, or, at least, to lukewarmness in religion; while some who were sincere Christians, exasperated by such reproaches, have sometimes expressed themselves unguardedly, and thereby afforded their enemies a handle to calumniate them. This, I imagine, has been the real source of that charge of infidelity, so often, and so unjustly brought against physicians."——"The study of medicine, of all others, should be the least suspected of leading to impiety. An intimate acquaintance with the works of nature raises the mind to the most sublime conceptions of the Supreme Being; and at the same time dilates the heart with the most pleasing views of Providence. The difficulties that necessarily attend all deep enquiries into a subject so disproportionate to the human faculties, should not be suspected

to

to surprise a physician, who, in his practice, is often involved in perplexity, even in subjects exposed to the examination of his senses."

"There are besides, some peculiar circumstances, in the profession of a physician, which should naturally dispose him to look beyond the present scene of things, and engage his heart on the side of religion. He has many opportunities of seeing people, once the gay and the happy, sunk in deep distress; sometimes devoted to a painful and lingering death; and sometimes struggling with the tortures of a distracted mind. Such afflictive scenes, one should imagine, might soften any heart, not dead to every feeling of humanity; and make it reverence that religion which alone can support the soul in the most complicated distresses; that religion, which teaches to enjoy life with cheerfulness, and to resign it with dignity."

The judicious and animated considerations which are here delivered, could proceed only from a mind actuated by the principles of virtue and religion. And I trust, the great majority of physicians have their feelings in unison with those of the amiable writer I have quoted. But there may be some who have been hardened to moral apathy, by the very causes which should excite benevolence and piety.

piety. It has been well remarked, by divines and metaphysicians, that *passive impressions* become progressively weaker by frequent recurrence; and that the heart is liable to grow callous to scenes of horror and distress, and even to the view of death itself. This law of nature is intended, by the wise and benignant author of our frame, to answer the most salutary purposes, by co-operating with another of equal, perhaps superior, force. For *active propensities* are formed, and gradually strengthened, by the like renewal of the circumstances which excite them. The love of goodness is thus rendered habitual; and rectitude of conduct is steadily and uniformly pursued, without struggle or perturbation.

The human character then attains the highest excellence, of which this probationary state is capable; and, perhaps, no profession is more favourable, than that of physic, to the formation of a mental constitution, which unites in it very high degrees of intellectual and moral vigour; because it calls forth the steady and unremitting exertions of benevolence, under the direction of cultivated reason; and, by opening a wider and wider sphere of duty, progressively augments their reciprocal energies. But the connection between the laws of of impression, and of habit, is not so determinate and necessary as to be wholly independent of the agent who is under their influence. By a perversion of the understanding and the will, they may be, and sometimes are, separated. The affections also, when the temperament is phlegmatic, subsist only in a languid state; and are too evanescent to produce a permanently correspondent frame of mind. If with this coldness of heart, a sceptical turn of thinking happen to be associated, either constitutionally or from the casualties of study and connections, virtuous principles will gradually decay; all the tender charities of life will soon be extinguished; a future state will be either disbelieved or regarded with indifference; and practical atheism will ensue, with the whole train of evils which result from a denial of the creative agency of God, or his divine administration. Allowing this to be an extreme, and barely possible case, a concession which I am solicitous to grant to my countrymen, notwithstanding what has been fatally experienced in a neighbouring kingdom; yet different gradations towards it may subsist, and the first step should be avoided with sedulous care. The countervailing power of religion is here essentially necessary, because nothing be-

 sides

sides can furnish motives to rectitude, of adequate dignity, weight and authority. To restore the impressions of piety which have been lost or impaired, without falling into the fervours of enthusiasm, or the gloom of superstition, may be an arduous task, a task that will require time and perseverance to accomplish. But the attainment will amply repay the labour, by the sweet satisfaction which a physician cannot fail to derive from the consciousness, that he exercises his profession under the inspection of a Being, who approves, and will reward every effort to acquire his favour by doing good to mankind. In his offices of humanity, he will feel an interest and elevation, of which those can have no conception who regard the human race, and consequently the sufferers under their care, not as the offspring of God, or as expectants of immortality, but as the creatures of a day, formed by the casual concourse, or the natural appetencies of atoms, and born only to perish. Such degrading and unhappy notions often spring from a love of paradox; a passion for novel hypothesis; ambition to be victorious in subtle disputation; and a contempt for established authority, accompanied, for the most part, with an implicit submission to empirics in science, who

who dogmatize most, when they assume the mask of scepticism. To the successful pursuit of truth it is necessary to bring a well-disciplined mind, modest and sober in its views, and uninfluenced not only by vulgar, but by philosophical prejudices, which are far more dangerous, because more plausible and fascinating. When subjects which relate to theology are investigated, reverence and humility should be associated with all our reasonings. No practice is more subversive of devotional sentiment, than that of carrying into religious discussions the licentiousness of thought and expression, which young physicians are too apt to indulge on medical topics. He who can suffer himself to treat his Maker with indifference and with levity, whether it be in utterance or in contemplation, will soon lose the religious impressions of reverence, gratitude and love; and his mind will then be prepared for the system of impiety and atheism, which of late have been so boldly promulgated under the imposing name of philosophy. Productions of this class should be shunned, even by those who are thoroughly grounded in rational faith; because familiarity with them can hardly fail to impair the moral sensibilities of the heart.

They are *evil communications*, which forcibly tend to *corrupt good manners*.

To the comprehensive view of a well-educated physician, the Divine Being will appear, with the fullest manifestation, in all without and all within him. Through the several kingdoms of nature, with which he is intimately acquainted, he traces every where design, intelligence, power, wisdom, and goodness. And in the frame of his own body, as well as in the constitution of his mental faculties, he finds especial reason to conclude, that above all the other works of the creation, *he is fearfully and wonderfully made.* The daily offices of his profession disclose to him irrefragable proofs of the providence and moral government of God.—Health, as consisting in the soundness and vigour of the bodily organs, and in their complete aptitude for exertion and enjoyment, is doubtless of inestimable consideration. But the occasional suspension of this blessing may be necessary to obviate the abuses to which it is liable; to evince its high value; to remedy the injuries it may have sustained; and to insure its future more permanent duration. A strong constitution is too often made subservient to sensuality, ebriety, and other licentious indulgences, which,

which, if not seasonably interrupted by the experience of *consequential suffering*, would prove destructive to the animal œconomy, and bring on premature decripetude or death. Diseases, under these circumstances, furnish a beneficial restraint, and preserve the mind from contamination; whilst they are often the remedies, which nature has kindlv provided, for the restoration of the vital functions. A good, which has been lost and beneficently restored, will be prized according to its high desert; and being cherished with assiduous care, will be prolonged and applied to its proper uses, in the great business of life. But sickness, it must be acknowledged, is not always remedial in its tendency; and frequently produces degrees of protracted languishment and pain, grievous to endure, and obstructive of those *active offices*, which, in his present sphere, man is called upon to perform. There are duties, however, of another class, not less essential to the improvement and excellence of his *moral* and *religious character:* And where is a school to be found, like the chamber of sickness for meekness, patience, resignation, gratitude, and devout trust in God? There pride is humbled; the angry passions subside; animosities cease; and the vanities of the world

world lose their bewitching attractions. False associations are there corrected; true estimates are formed; and whilst the *passive virtues* are cultivated in the suffering individual, all who minister to him have their best dispositions exercised, and improved. Tenderness, humanity, sympathy, friendship, and domestic love, on such occasions, find that sphere which is peculiarly adapted to their exertion; and all the softer charities derive from these sources, their highest refinements. *(a)*

Rational theism leads the mind, by fair and necessary induction, to extend its views to revelation. He who has discovered the divine wisdom, power, and goodness, through the various works of creation, will feel a solicitude to make farther advances in sacred knowledge; and the more profoundly he venerates the author of his being, the more earnest will he be to become acquainted with his will; with the means of conciliating his favour; with the duration of his own existence; and with his future destination. Several distinguished characters in the heathen world have, in a very explicit manner, testified the truth of this observation. Suffice it to state only the following remarkable passages from Plato: "A divine revelation is

" necessary

(a) See A Father's Instructions, Part III. page 312, 9th edition.

"necessary to explain the true worship of God "—to add authority to moral precepts—to "assist our best endeavours in a virtuous course "—to fix the future rewards and punishments "of virtuous and vicious conduct—and to "point out some acceptable expiation for "sin." He introduces Socrates, assuring Alcibiades, "that in a future time a divine "person will appear, who, in pure love to "man, shall remove all darkness from his "mind, and instruct him how to offer his prayers "and praises in the most acceptable way to "the Divine Being." The privileges which this intelligent and amiable philosopher ardently looked for, we happily enjoy. Christianity has brought life and immortality to light: And the gospel is the sacred charter of our expected inheritance of felicity. To regard with indifference what is so momentous, is the grossest folly; to be dissatisfied with its evidence argues the want of discernment and of candour; and to reject it, without deliberate and conscientious investigation, is a high degree of impiety: The appeal, however, must finally be made to the judgment of every individual. And we may humbly hope, that he who *knoweth our frame*, will pity intellectual infirmity, and pardon involuntary error.

Note

Note XIII. *Chap.* II. *Sect.* XXXI.

UNION IN CONSULTATION OF SENIOR AND JUNIOR PHYSICIANS.

"Heat and vivacity in age," says Bacon, "is an excellent composition for business. Young men are fitter to invent than to judge, fitter for execution than for counsel, and fitter for new projects than for settled business; for the experience of age in things that fall within the compass of it, directeth them, but in new things abuseth them. The errors of young men are the ruin of business; but the errors of aged men amount but to this, that more might have been done or sooner. Young men, in the conduct and manage of actions, embrace more than they can hold, stir more than they can quiet, fly to the end without consideration of the means and degrees, pursue some few principles which they have chanced upon absurdly, care not to innovate, which draws unknown inconveniences; use extreme remedies at first, and that which doubleth all errors, will not acknowledge or retract them, like an unruly horse that will neither stop nor turn. Men of age object too much, consult too long, adventure too little, repent too soon, and seldom

dom drive business home to the full period, but content themselves with a mediocrity of success. Certainly it is good to compound employments of both; for that will be good for the present, because the virtues of either age may correct the defects of both; and good for succession, that young men may be learners, while men in age are actors. And lastly, good for extern accidents, because authority followeth old men, and favour and popularity youth: But for the moral part, perhaps youth will have the pre-eminence, as age hath for the politick.—Bacon's Essay of Youth and Age."

Note XIV. *Chap.* II. *Sect.* XXXII.

RETIREMENT FROM PRACTICE.

The following letters afford so admirable a comment on the rule to which this note refers, that it would be a false and unjustifiable delicacy not to lay them before the reader. I shall copy them without abridgment, because they present at once a striking display of Dr. Heberden's nice sense of honour and probity; of the peculiar urbanity of his manners; and of the vigour of his intellect at a very advanced period of life. His commendations of

this

this little work, I may be allowed to confess, are gratifying to my feelings; though I am sensible of the partiality from which they flow. But the partiality of a character, dignified by science and virtue, is itself an honour.

Copy of a Letter from William Heberden, M. D. F. R. S. &c. &c.

Dear Sir, Windsor, 28 August, 1794.

It is owing to my distance from London, that I have not sooner made my acknowledgments, and returned my thanks for your very obliging letter. Your being able to resume the work you had in hand, makes me hope that your good principles, with the aid of time, have greatly recovered your mind from what you must have suffered on occasion of the great loss in your family; and your attention in the further prosecution of it, will powerfully assist in perfectly restoring your tranquillity. What you have already communicated to the public, with so much just applause, shews you to be peculiarly well qualified for drawing up a Code of Medical Ethics, by the just sense you have of your duties as a man, and by the masterly knowledge of your profession as a physician. I hope

hope it will not be long before the sheets already printed come to my hands; and I return you many thanks for intending to favor me with a sight of them.

The pleasure of a visit from one of Dr. Haygarth's merit, whom I have long known and esteemed, would probably give me spirits, and make him think me less broken than I am. I have entered my 85th year; and when I retired, a few years ago, from the practice of physic, I trust it was not from a wish to be idle, which no man capable of being usefully employed has a right to be, but because I was willing to give over, before my presence of thought, judgment, and recollection were so impaired, that I could not do justice to my patients. It is more desirable for a man to do this a little too soon, than a little too late; for the chief danger is on the side of not doing it soon enough. I am, my dear sir,

With great esteem and regard,

Your affectionate, humble servant,

W. HEBERDEN.

From the Same.

DEAR SIR, Pall Mall, 15th October, 1794.

BY the mistake, or neglect of the person left in my house in London (to which

 I am

I am just returned) your Code of Medical Ethics had been sent thither some time before I was made acquainted with it. I have read it, and do not wonder, that nothing could be found by me, or by any one to add or alter, after a work of this kind had passed through the hands of one so much master of the subject; and who had taken no little time to consider it, and to make the proper improvements. I am confident that the same might be said of them, were I to read the two chapters which remain to be finished. If your judicious advice and rules were duly observed, they would greatly contribute to support the dignity of the profession, and the peace and comfort of the professors. There has lately been established, in several of the London hospitals, a plan of courses of lectures in all the branches of knowledge useful to a student in physic. Such plans, if rightly executed, as I have no reason to doubt they will be, must make London a school of physic, superior to most in Europe. The experience afforded in an hospital, will keep down the luxuriance of plausible theories. Many such have been delivered in lectures, by celebrated teachers, with great applause; but the students, though perfectly masters of them, not having corrected them with what nature exhibits

exhibits in an hospital, have found themselves more at a loss in the cure of a patient, than an elder apprentice of an apothecary. I please myself with thinking, that the method of teaching the art of healing, is becoming every day more conformable to what reason and nature require; that the errors introduced by superstition and false philosophy are gradually retreating; and that medical knowledge, as well as all other dependent upon observation and experience, is continually increasing in the world. The present race of physicians are possessed of several most important rules of practice, utterly unknown to the ablest in former ages, not excepting Hippocrates himself, or even Æsculapius.

I am, dear sir,
Your affectionate, humble servant,
W. Heberden.

It is an observation of Bacon, that letters written by wise men, are the best of all human works. To these admirable communications, I shall, therefore, take the liberty of subjoining the extract of one, equally interesting and of similar import, from another Nestor in medicine; who has long and justly held the first rank amongst his brethren, for classical taste, elegance

elegance of style, and professional erudition. "I have lately," says Sir George Baker, in a letter, dated Richmond, August 11th, 1802, "been in the habit of spending much of my "time in this place; avoiding, when possible, "all medical employment. Many months "have passed since Dr. Haygarth took so fa-"vorable a measure of me: I will not, how-"ever, trouble you with an account of the in-"firmities and privations incident to my time "of life. Be it sufficient to say, that I am con-"tented with the fare that I have met with; "and hope to retire from the feast of life *uti* "*conviva satur.*"

Note XV. *Chap.* IV. *Sect.* II.

PARTIAL INSANITY, WITH GENERAL INTELLIGENCE. LUCID INTERVAL.

Sir Matthew Hale, in his *Historia Placitorum Coronæ*, C. iv. has stated, that "There "is a partial insanity of mind; and a total in-"sanity. The former is either in respect to "things, *quoad hoc vel illud insanire;* some "persons that have a competent use of reason "in respect to some subjects, are yet under a "particular *dementia*, in respect to some par-"ticular

"ticular discourses, subjects, or applications; "or else it is particular in respect of degrees; "and this is the condition of very many, espe- "cially melancholy persons, who, for the most "part, discover their defect in excessive fears and "griefs, and yet are not wholly destitute of the "use of reason, and this partial insanity seems "not to excuse them in the committing of any "offence for its matter capital, for doubtless "most persons that are felons of themselves, "and others, are under a degree of partial in- "sanity, when they commit these offences."— "The person that is absolutely mad for a day, "killing a man in that distemper, is equally "not guilty, as if he were mad without inter- "mission. But such persons as have their "lucid intervals (which ordinarily happen be- "tween the full and change of the moon) in "such intervals have usually at least a compe- "tent use of reason, and crimes committed by "them in these intervals are of the same nature, "and subject to the same punishment, as if they "had no such deficiency, nay, the alienations "and contracts made by them in such intervals, "are obliging to their heirs and executors."

Partial insanity and general intelligence may subsist, in various degrees and proportions to each other, in different persons; and even in in the same person at different times. If Socrates had lived at this period, and had not only professed himself to be governed by the influences of a familiar spirit, or dæmon, but had, also, uniformly regulated his conversation and actions by this persuasion, he would have been justly chargeable with derangement of mind, notwithstanding the profound wisdom which he displayed in his instructions concerning morals, and the conduct of life. Lord Herbert, of Cherbury, was highlv distinguished both for talents and erudition: But having unfortunately adopted prejudices against Christianity, he wrote an elaborate work entitled, *De Veritate, prout distinguitur a Revelatione;* and knowing it would meet with much opposition, he remained some time in anxious suspense about the publication of it. Providence, however, as he informs us in his own biographical memoirs, kindly interposed, and determined his wavering resolutions. "Being "thus doubtful in my chamber, one fair day "in the summer, my casement being open to-"wards the south, and no wind stirring, I "took my book *De Veritate* in my hand, and "kneeling on my knees, devoutly said, *O thou "eternal God, I am not satisfied enough whe-"ther I shall publish this book; if it be to thy*

"glory,

"*glory, I beseech thee give me some sign from* "*heaven; if not, I shall suppress it.* I had no "sooner spoken these words, but a loud, though "yet gentle noise, came from the heavens, "which did so comfort and chear me, that "I took my petition as granted, and that I "had the sign I demanded; whereupon also "I resolved to print my book." This was not a temporary delusion of the imagination, but continued a permanent object of belief through life. And the impression was more extraordinary, and more indicative of an unsound mind, because Lord Herbert's chief argument against Christianity is, the improbability that Heaven shall reveal its laws *only to a portion of the earth.* For how could he, who doubted of a *partial*, confide in an *individual* revelation? Or is it possible that he could rationally think his book of sufficient importance to extort a declaration of the divine will, when the interest and happiness of a fourth part of mankind were deemed, by him, objects inadequate to the like display of goodness.*

The history of the Rev. Simon Browne, still more remarkably exemplifies the union of vi-

* See Walpole's Catalogue of royal and noble Authors; also Percival's Mor. and Lit. Diss. p. 82.

gour and imbecility, of rectitude and perversion in the same understanding. The loss of his wife, and of his only son, so powerfully affected him, that he desisted from the duties of his clerical function, and could not be persuaded to join in any act of worship to the Deity, either public or private. He "conceived "that Almighty God, by a singular instance "of divine power, had, in a gradual man-"ner, annihilated in him the thinking sub-"stance, and utterly divested him of conscious-"ness: That though he retained the human "shape, and the faculty of speaking, in a "manner that appeared to others rational, he "had all the while no more notion of what "he said than a parrot. And, very consist-"ently with this, he looked upon himself as "no longer a moral agent, a subject of reward "or punishment." In this conviction he continued, with very little variation, to the close of life. Yet, whilst under the influence of this strange phrensy, his faculties, in all other respects, appeared to be in full vigour. He applied himself with ardour to his studies; and was so acute a disputant, that his friends were wont to say, *he could reason as if possessed of two souls*. Indeed, both his imagination and his judgment were so improved,

as

as to surpass the state in which they subsisted during his perfect sanity.*

In J. J. Rousseau, we have a most interesting example of morbid sensibility and depraved imagination, combined with extensive knowledge and pre-eminent genius. It is said by Madam de Stael, in her Reflections on his Character and Writings, that "sometimes he "would part with you, with all his former af-"fection; but if an expression had escaped "you, which might bear an unfavourable "construction; he would recollect it, exa-"mine it, exaggerate it, perhaps dwell upon "it for a month, and conclude by a total "breach with you. Hence it was, that there "was scarce a possibility of undeceiving him; "for the light which broke in upon him at "once, was not sufficient to efface the wrong "impressions which had taken place so gra-"dually in his mind. It was extremely dif-"ficult too to continue long on an intimate "footing with him. A word, a gesture, fur-"nished him with matter of profound medi-"tation; he connected the most trifling cir-"cumstances, like so many mathematical pro-

 "positions,

* See Biog. Britan. Art. Simon Browne.

" positions, and conceived his conclusion to be " supported by the evidence of demonstration.*

I have hazarded an opinion in the text, contrary to what, I believe, is usually adopted by lawyers, that there may be cases of partial insanity with a high degree of general intelligence, in which the individual ought not to be precluded from the privilege of making a last will and testament. To deny the testamentary qualification to one, who, notwithstanding some false predominant conception, has been held capable of managing his concerns with discretion, and whose bequests discover no traces of a disturbed imagination, or unsound judgment, seems to be inconsistent both with wisdom and with natural justice. Such a person, I presume, is capable of acquiring property by legacy, by bargain, by transfer, by industry, or by office: And he is not prohibited, during life, from giving or expending possessions thus obtained. Why then does the law deprive him of the right of bequeathing after death, that which he might have dispensed, when alive, without controul? Whatever be the opinion which a medical practitioner

* The reader is referred to the Elements of the Philosophy of the Human Mind, Sect. V. by Professor Dugald Stewart, for some admirable remarks on the evils which result from an ill-regulated imagination.

titioner may have entertained, concerning the capacity or incapacity for making a will of one under these circumstances, it can hardly be necessary to observe, that his evidence, when called for in a course of legal enquiry, should be delivered explicitly, and without any bias from his pre-conceptions. On the point litigated, it is the exclusive province of the judge and jury to decide, after a full investigation of the case.

To determine the existence of a LUCID INTERVAL in the *delirium* of *fever*; or in the more permanent alienation of mind which constitutes *insanity*, the testimony of a physician is sometimes required, in courts of law. It will be incumbent on him, therefore, to possess a clear and definite opinion on the subject, founded both on the nature of the malady, and the state of the patient. The cessation of febrile delirium is not difficult to ascertain; because the rational faculties being unimpaired by a short suspension, at once manifest their renewal by signs which cannot be misunderstood. But the complete remission of madness, is only to be decided by reiterated and attentive observation. Every action, and even gesture of the patient should be sedulously watched; and he should be drawn

drawn into conversations, at different times, that may insensibly lead him to develope the false impressions under which he labours. He should also be employed, occasionally, in business, or offices connected with, and likely to renew his wrong associations. If these trials produce no recurrence of insanity, he may, with full assurance, be regarded as legally *compos mentis*, during such period; even though he should relapse, a short time afterward, into his former malady.

Note XVI. *Chap.* IV. *Sect.* XIII.

DUELLING.

In the usages of the ancient Germans, evident traces of DUELLING may be discovered. But it was employed by them either as an appeal to the justice, or to the prescience of the gods. Velleius Paterculus informs us, that questions, decided amongst the Romans by legal trial, were terminated amongst the Germans by arms or judicial combat.* Tacitus describes it as a species of divination, by which the future events of important wars were explored. A captive from the enemy was compelled

* Vellei Patercul. lib. II. cap. cxviii.

pelled to fight with a man selected from their own nation. Each was accoutred with his proper weapons; and the presage of success was determined by the issue of the battle.* A law is quoted by Stiernhoök, which shews, that judicial combat was, at first, appropriated to points respecting personal character, and that it was only subsequently extended to criminal cases, and to questions relative to property. The terms of the law are, "If any man shall say to another these reproachful words, 'you are not a man equal to other men,' or, 'you have not the heart of a man,' and the other shall reply 'I am a man as good as you,' let them meet on the highway. If he who first gave offence appear, and the person absent himself, let the latter be deemed worse than he was called; let him not be admitted to give evidence in judgment either for man or woman, and let him not have the privilege of making a testament. If the person offended appear, and he who gave the offence be absent, let him call upon the other thrice with a loud voice, and make a mark upon the earth, and then let him who absented himself be

* Vide Tacit. de Situ, Morib. et Populis Germaniæ, Sect. X.

be deemed infamous, because he uttered words which he durst not support If both shall appear properly armed, and the person offended shall fall in the combat, let a half compensation be paid for his death. But if the person who gave the offence shall fall, let it be imputed to his own rashness. The petulance of his tongue hath been fatal to him. Let him lie in the field without any compensation being made for his death.*

Montesquieu, on the authority of Beaumanoir, whom he quotes with great respect, deduces the rise and formation of the articles, relative to the point of honour, from the following particular judicial usages. The accuser declared, in the presence of the judge, that such a person had committed such an action: The accused made answer that *he lied*, upon which the judge gave orders for the duel. Thus it became an established rule, that whenever the lie was given to a person, it was incumbent on him to fight. *Gentlemen* combatted on horseback, completely armed. *Villeins* fought on foot, and with bastons. The baston, therefore, was regarded as an instrument of affront, because to strike a man with it was to treat him as a villein.

* Lex Uplandica apud Stiern.—Robertson's History of Charles V. vol. I. Note 22.

villein. For the like reason, a box on the ear, or blow on the face, was deemed a contumely, to be expiated with blood; since villeins alone were liable to receive such disgraceful blows, as it was peculiar to them to fight with their heads uncovered.*

Practices like these were so congenial to the proud and martial spirit of the times, as well as to the superstition which prevailed, that they became universal throughout Europe. But it is evident that they could not fail to subvert the regular course of justice, diminish the authority of government, and violate the sacred ordinances of the church. For the clergy uniformly remonstrated against, and even anathematized them, as adverse to christianity; and the civil power frequently interposed, to set bounds to usages, which its authority was too feeble to suppress. Henry I. of England, in the twelfth century, prohibited trial by combat, in all questions concerning property of small value. Louis VII. of France issued an edict to the same effect. St. Louis, who was a distinguished legislator, considering the rude age in which he reigned, attempted a more perfect jurisprudence, by substituting trial by evidence, in place of that by

 combat.

* See Montesquieu, Liv. XXVIII. C. XX.

combat. And afterwards it became the policy of every monarch, who possessed power or talents, to explode these relics of Gothic barbarism. By degrees the practice became less and less frequent; courts of judicature acquired an ascendancy; law was studied as a science, and administered with great regularity; and the ferocious manners of the inhabitants of Europe yielded to the arts of peace, and to the benefits of social and civilized life. But an event occurred, in the year 1528, which both revived the practice of single combat, and gave a new form to it, more absurd and fatal. The political and personal enmity, which subsisted between the Emperor Charles V. and Francis I., led the former to commission the French herald, sent to him with a denunciation of war, to acquaint his sovereign, that he should from that time consider him not only as a base violator of public faith, but as a stranger to the honour and probity of a gentleman. Francis instantly sent back the herald, with a *cartel* of defiance, giving the Emperor *the lie*, and challenging him to single combat. Charles accepted the challenge; but it being impracticable to settle the preliminaries, this romantic and ridiculous enterprize of course was never accomplished. The transaction,

action, however, excited such universal attention, and reflected so much splendour and dignity on this novel mode of single combat, that every gentleman thought himself entitled, and even bound in honour to draw his sword, and to demand satisfaction of his adversary, for affronts trivial, and even imaginary.* The best blood in Christendom was shed; personages of the first distinction were devoted to death; the ease, the familiarity, and the confidence of private intercourse were interrupted; and war itself was hardly more destructive to life, and to its dearest enjoyments, than this fatal and seductive frenzy.†

 Evils

* See Robertson's History of Charles V. Book V.

† The History of Lord Herbert of Cherbury, who lived in the reigns of Queen Elizabeth and James I., fully exemplifies the folly and danger of adopting false principles of honour. During the abode of this romantic nobleman, at the Duke of Montmorenci's, about twenty-four miles from Paris, it happened, one evening, that a daughter of the Duchess de Ventadour, of about ten or eleven years of age, went to walk in the meadows, with his lordship, and several other gentlemen and ladies. The young lady wore a knot of ribband on her head, which a French chevalier snatched away, and fastened to his hatband. He was desired to return it, but refused. The lady then requested Lord Herbert to recover it for her. A race ensued; and the chevalier, finding

Evils of such magnitude required adequate remedies; and all the terrors of law were every where exerted to repress them. But they have hitherto been employed in vain. Nor is it likely that sanguinary punishments will prevail, because the dread of such punishment would be deemed equally dishonourable with the fear of death, in the chances of combat. A heavy fine, strictly levied, would operate with greater force, on some of the most active principles of the human mind: And if it amounted to half, or one third of the convicted person's fortune, such portion being placed in chancery, for the benefit of his heirs or children, this privation would not only extend to his comforts and accommodations, but would be felt as a species of infamy, by

finding himself likely to be overtaken, made a sudden turn, and was about to deliver his prize to the young lady, when Lord Herbert seized his arm, and cried out, "I "give it you." "Pardon me," said the lady, "it is he "who gives it me." "Madam," replied Lord Herbert, "I will not contradict you, but if the chevalier do not "acknowledge that I constrain him to give the ribband, "I will fight with him." And the next day, he sent him a challenge, "being bound thereto," says he, "by the "oath taken when I was made knight of the bath." See the Life of Lord Herbert, of Cherbury; also Percival's Moral and Lit. Dissert. p. 299, second edit.

by depriving him of the means of maintaining his rank and station in life. Lord Verulam has proposed the following remedy for duelling; which, if effectual with men of quality, would soon disgrace the practice amongst those of inferior degree: "The fountain of honour is the "king; and his aspect, and the access to his "person continueth honour in life; and to be "banished from his presence is one of the "greatest eclipses of honour that can be; if "his Majesty shall be pleased, that when "this court shall censure any of these offences, in persons of eminent quality, to "add this out of his own power and discipline, "that those persons shall be banished and excluded from his court for certain years, and "the courts of his Queen and Prince, I think "there is no man that hath any good blood "in him, will commit an act that shall cast "him into that darkness, that he may not behold his sovereign's face."* This proposal of Lord Verulam seems to receive some confirmation from a story, related by Lord Shaftsbury, in his Characteristicks.† "A certain gallant of our court, being asked by his friends, why one of his established character for courage

* Bacon's Works, Vol. II. page 516.

† Vol. I. Sect. III. page 273.

rage and good-sense, would answer the challenge of a coxcomb, replied, "that for his "*own sex* he could safely trust their judgment: "But how could he appear at night before the "*maids of honour?*"

Thus the principle, on which duelling is founded, is now neither an appeal to the justice of heaven, nor an expression of resentment for wrong sustained; but generally a mere punctilio of honour, which would affix a *stigma* on the character for courage of him, who omits to offer, and on the opponent who declines the acceptance of a challenge. Hence forgiveness of injury, and reparation from the consciousness of having committed it, those noble sentiments of just and generous minds, are wholly precluded in the intercourse of fashionable life.

A very able moralist, whom I have often quoted with peculiar satisfaction, has reduced the question concerning duelling, as now practised, to this single point: Whether a regard for our own reputation is, or is not, sufficient to justify the taking away the life of another. "A sense of shame," says he, "is so much "torture; and no relief presents itself, other-"wise than by an attempt upon the life of our "adversary. What then? The distress which "men

" men suffer by the want of money is often-
" times extreme, and no resource can be dis-
" covered but that of removing a life, which
" stands between the distressed person and his
" inheritance. The motive in this case is as
" urgent, and the means much the same, as
" in the former; yet this case finds no advo-
" cates."

" For the army, where the point of honour
" is cultivated with exquisite attention and re-
" finement," continues the same excellent writer, " I would establish a court of honour,
" with a power of awarding those submissions
" and acknowledgments, which it is gene-
" rally the object of a challenge to obtain;
" and it might grow into a fashion, with per-
" sons of rank of all professions to refer their
" quarrels to the same tribunal."*

An institution, like the one thus forcibly recommended by Dr. Paley, might probably have prevented the late fatal duel between Colonel Montgomery and Captain M'Namara. The address of the latter to the gentlemen of the jury gives just grounds for this opinion, and claims on that account the attention of the legislature. " Gentlemen," said he, " I am a cap-
" tain

* Dr. Paley's Principles of Moral Philosophy, Chap. IX.

" tain of the British navy. My character you " can only hear from others; but to maintain " any character, in that station, I must be re- " spected. When called upon to lead others into " honourable dangers, I must not be supposed " to be a man who had sought safety, by sub- " mitting to what custom has taught others to " consider as a disgrace. I am not presuming " to urge any thing against the laws of God, " or of this land. I know that, in the eye of " religion and reason, obedience to the law, " though against the general feelings of the " world, is the first duty, and ought to be the " rule of action: but in putting a construc- " tion upon my motives, so as to ascertain the " quality of my actions, you will make allow- " ances for my situation.* In referring to the foregoing disastrous case, it is proper to notice, that a surgeon of considerable eminence, who attended on the field of combat in his *professional capacity*, was on this account arrested, and sent to Newgate, by a warrant from the civil magistrate, as a *principal* in the alledged murder, having been present at the duel, and antecedently privy to it. Nor was he liberated from

* Courier, April 23, 1803.

from prison till the grand jury had rejected the indictment.

It has recently been stated, in one of the periodical prints, that a law to prevent duelling was passed in the general assembly of North Carolina during their last session, by which it was enacted, "That no person sending, accepting, or being the bearer of a "challenge, for the purpose of fighting a duel, "even though no death should ensue, shall "ever after be eligible to any office of trust, "power, or profit in the state, any pardon "or reprieve notwithstanding: And that the "said person shall further be liable to be indicted, and on conviction shall forfeit and "pay the sum of one hundred pounds to the "use of the state. And if any one fight a "duel, by which either of the parties shall be "killed, then the survivor on conviction thereof, shall suffer death without benefit of clergy; "and the seconds shall be considered as accessaries before the fact, and likewise suffer "death."*

I shall insert the following communication from my late venerable friend Dr. Benjamin Franklin, on the subject of duelling, because

* Courier, March 9th, 1803.

cause the deliberate opinion of a man, peculiarly distinguished by perspicacity, soundness of judgment, and extensive knowledge of the world, cannot fail to be interesting to the reader. The letter was written in the 79th year of his age, and evinces the same vein of humour which characterized him through life. A few passages are omitted, being merely complimentary and personal.

Passy, near Paris, July 17, 1784.

DEAR SIR,

I received, yesterday, by Mr. White, your kind letter of May 11th, with the most agreeable present of your new book. I read it all before I slept. *

It is astonishing that the murderous practice of duelling, which you so justly condemn, should continue so long in vogue. Formerly when duels were used to determine law-suits, from an opinion that Providence would, in every instance, favour truth and right with victory, they were more excusable. At present they decide nothing. A man says something, which another tells him is a lie. They fight; but whichever is killed, the point in dispute

dispute remains unsettled. To this purpose they have a pleasant little story here: A gentleman, in a coffee-house, desired another to sit farther from him.—Why so?—Because, Sir, you smell offensively.—That is an affront, and you must fight me. I will fight you if you insist upon it: But I do not see how that will mend the matter. For if you kill me I shall smell too; and if I kill you, you will smell, if possible, worse than you do at present:—How can such miserable sinners as we are, entertain so much pride as to conceive that every offence against our imagined honour merits death? These petty princes, in their own opinion, would call that sovereign a tyrant, who should put one of them to death for a little uncivil language, though pointed at his sacred person. Yet every one of them makes himself judge in his own cause; condemns the offender without a jury, and undertakes himself to be the executioner.

Our friend Mr. Vaughan may, perhaps, communicate to you some conjectures of mine, relating to the cold of last winter, which I sent him in return for the observations on cold of professor Wilson. If he should, and you think them worthy so much notice, you may shew them to your philosophical society, to which I

 wish

wish all imaginable success. Their rules seem to me excellent.

With sincere and great esteem, I have the honour to be, your most obedient,

and most humble servant,

B. FRANKLIN.

Note XVII. *Chap.* IV *Sect.* XVI.

PUNISHMENT OF THE CRIME OF RAPE.

THE atrocity of this crime appears to have been variously estimated at different periods, and in different countries; if we may judge from the diversity of punishments inflicted on the perpetrators of it. The reader will find a copious and interesting enumeration of them, in a folio volume, entitled, *A View of Ancient Laws against Immorality and Profaneness, by John Disney, M. A. Cambridge printed,* 1729. I would refer him also to the *Principles of Penal Law*, by Mr. Eden, now Lord Auckland. As both these valuable works are out of print, a few extracts from each may form an acceptable addition to the present note.

The Burgundian laws provided, that if the young woman carried off, returned to her parents

rents actually corrupted, the offender should pay six times her price, or legal valuation; and also a mulct of twelve shillings. If he had not wherewithal to pay these sums, he should be given up to her parents, or near relations, to take their revenge of him in what way they pleased.

By the law of Æthelbert, the first Christian king of Kent, it was enacted, that if any person take a young woman by force, he shall pay her parent, or guardian, fifty shillings; and shall make a farther composition for her ransom. If she were espoused, he shall compensate the husband by an additional payment of twenty shillings. But if she were with child, the augmented fine shall be five and thirty shillings, and fifteen more to the king.

There is an ordinance of king Alfred, for the punishment of Rapes, committed upon country wenches who were servants, an offence which may be supposed to have been prevalent at that time. Is is delivered in the following terms: " *Si quis Coloni mancipium ad stuprum comminetur* 5 *Sol. Colono emendet, et* 60 *Sol. Mulctæ loco. Si Servus Servam ad stuprum coegerit, compenset hoc Virgâ suâ virili. Si quis puellam teneræ ætatis ad illicitum concubitum comminetur, eodem modo puniatur*

puniatur quo ille, qui adultæ servæ hoc fecerit."

By the Welsh laws of Prince Hoel Dha, if two women were walking together without other company, and violence was offered to either or both of them, it was not punishable as a rape; but if they had a third person with them, they might claim their full legal redress. If the perpetrator of a rape, being accused, confessed the fact, besides full satisfaction to the woman, he was to answer for the crime to his sovereign, by the present of a silver stand as high as the king's mouth, and as thick as his middle finger, with a gold cup upon it, so large as to contain what he could take off at one draught, and as thick as the nail of a country fellow who had worked at the plough seven years. If the offender was not able to make such a present, *virilia membra amittat.*

Sir Edward Coke states this offence as a felony at the common law, which had a punishment, "under such a condition as no other "felony had the like." The criminal was adjudged *amittere oculos, quibus virginem concupivit; amittere etiam testiculos, qui calorem stupri induxerunt.*

In the ancient law of England, exclusive of the punishment inflicted on the criminal, his

his horse, greyhound and hawk, were also subjected to great corporal infamy: But the woman who was the sufferer, might prevent all the penalties, if, before judgment, she demanded the offender for her husband. The Roman law was in the same spirit. "*Rapta* "*raptoris, aut mortem, aut indotatas nup-* "*tias optet*;" upon which there arose what was thought a doubtful case, "*Una nocte* "*quidam duas rapuit, altera mortem optat,* "*altera nuptias.*"

Note XVIII. *Chap.* IV. *Sect.* XVI.

UNCERTAINTY IN THE EXTERNAL SIGNS OF RAPE.

I have been favoured by Mr. Ward, one of the surgeons to the Manchester Infirmary, with the following particulars of the case, to which this note refers.

"Jane Hampson, aged four, was admitted an out-patient of the Infirmary, February 11th, 1791. The female organs were highly inflamed, sore, and painful; and it was stated by the mother, that the child was as well as usual till the preceding day, when she complained of pain in making water. This induced

duced the mother to examine the parts affected, when she was surprized to find the appearances above described. The child had slept, two or three nights, in the same bed with a boy, fourteen years old; and had complained that morning of having been hurt by him very much in the night."

"Leeches, and other external applications, together with appropriate internal remedies, were prescribed: But the debility increased, and on the 20th of February the child died. The coroner's inquest was taken, previously to which the body was inspected, and the abdominal and thoracic *viscera* were found to have been free from disease. The circumstances above related having been proved to the satisfaction of the jury, and being corroborated by the opinion I gave, that the child's death was occasioned by external violence, a verdict of murder was returned against the boy with whom she had slept. A warrant was, therefore, issued to apprehend him; but he had absconded, a circumstance which was considered as a confirmation of his guilt, when added to the circumstantial evidence alledged against him."

"Not many weeks had elapsed, however, before several similar cases occurred, in which there

there was no reason to suspect that external violence had been offered; and some in which it was absolutely certain that no such injury could have taken place. A few of the patients died; though from the novelty and fatal tendency of the disease, more than common attention was paid to them. I was then convinced that I had been mistaken, in attributing Jane Hampson's death to external violence; and I informed the coroner of the reasons which produced this change of opinion. The testimony I gave was designedly made public; and the friends of the boy hearing of it, prevailed upon him to surrender himself."

"When he was called to the bar at Lancaster, the judge informed the jury, that the evidence adduced was not sufficient to convict him; that it would give rise to much indelicate discussion if they proceeded on the trial; and that he hoped, therefore, they would acquit him without calling any witnesses. With this request the jury immediately complied."

"The preceding narrative may teach the young surgeon to act with great circumspection, when called upon to give an opinion in cases which are involved in any degree of obscurity. It behoves him to consider well the important duty he has to discharge both to an individual,

 and

and to the community: And that he makes himself responsible for the consequences which may result from the influence of his judgment on the minds of the jury."

Note XIX. *Chap.* IV. *Sect.* XVIII.

THE SMOKE FROM LARGE WORKS A NUISANCE.

THE smoke issuing from large works, without any arsenical or other poisonous impregnation, may prove a great annoyance to the neighbourhood in which they are situated: And the proprietors should be compelled, by law, to diminish this evil, as much as possible, by the adoption of the improved methods of burning fuel, which have been lately invented. But it may be doubted whether the sooty matter, sublimed by the combustion of pit-coal, be so injurious, as is commonly supposed, to the animal œconomy, unless it should subsist in the atmosphere, in a very extraordinary degree of accumulation. The inhabitants of Coal-brook-Dale, who live in a narrow valley, where the air is almost constantly loaded with vapours from numerous furnaces, employed in the smelting of iron, are not, as I have been informed, peculiarly subject to pulmonary affections.

fections. And the people of Birmingham, Sheffield, Newcastle, and Manchester, towns which are often enveloped in smoke, from the nature of their respective manufactures, seem to suffer no abridgment in the general duration of life, as it subsists in crowded places, which can be ascribed exclusively to this cause. Hoffmann maintains, that the fumes of pit-coal are not injurious to health, in the ordinary modes of exposure to them: And Caspar Neumann confirms this testimony, by his experience and observation during a long residence in London.*

In mentioning Coalbrook-Dale, I might have stated the following fact, as corroborating the observation above advanced. A few years ago, a lady, accompanied by her husband, undertook a journey for the recovery of health, after a severe attack of asthma, to which she was often incident. The route lay through Coalbrook-Dale; and they arrived there on Sunday evening, about eight o'clock; when all the fires were fresh lighted for working the furnaces. A thick smoke pervaded the whole valley; and the gentleman was

 alarmed

* See Neumann's Chemical Works, by Lewis, page 246, 4to.

alarmed with the danger, which his wife incurred, of suffocation. But, to his surprize and satisfaction, she experienced no difficulty of breathing; and passed the night, inhaling the gross vapours with which she was surrounded, without present inconvenience or subsequent injury. May it be supposed that the sooty matter undergoes a decomposition in the lungs, by which it becomes capable of absorption, and innoxious to the animal œconomy? For the accumulation of it, as a solid substance, in the bronchial vesicles, could hardly fail to occasion immediate and permanent evils. It will, however, be alledged, that travellers breathe whole days in dusty roads, and yet experience no lasting bad effects. The case of masons, who are sometimes incident to hæmoptoe and pulmonary consumption, is widely different, as the particles, which they draw in by respiration, are large and angular.

Conceiving it to be of importance to obtain full and precise information, relative to the effects of smoke in Coalbrook-Dale, I wrote on this subject to Mr. Edwards, an eminent surgeon

surgeon who is settled there, from whom I have been favoured with the following judicious answer:

"I have never observed that asthmas, and "other pulmonic affections, are more frequent "in the Dale than elsewhere, but rather the "contrary; as I have been told, that the smoke "of London agrees better with some asthmatic "persons, than the keen country air. Old "colliers, indeed, and such as work in iron, "stone-mines, and lime-rocks, are very subject, "in the decline of life, to coughs and short-"ness of breath, especially hard drinkers; but "in other respects the inhabitants are remark-"ably healthy, and the principal part of the "practice is surgery, the smoke arising from "coal and iron not being so prejudicial as from "the copper-works, in Cornwal and other "parts. Such colliers and miners as are trou-"bled with coughs, &c. always ascribe it to "the dust arising in getting the coal or mi-"neral, and from the smoke in the burning "of lime, for which they take frequent eme-"tics and purges."

Coalbrook-Dale, June 18, 1803.

Note XX. *Page* 117.

DISCOURSE ON HOSPITAL DUTIES; BY THE REV. THO. B. PERCIVAL, LL. B.

THIS Anniversary Discourse was addressed to the gentlemen of the faculty; the officers; the clergy; and the trustees of the Infirmary, at Liverpool, for the benefit of the charity; and I believe was highly approved by the judicious audience, before whom it was delivered. As the preacher assumed topics of exhortation, not before adopted by divines on such occasions, it may be proper to state, that he was peculiarly qualified, from his knowledge of the polity of hospitals, to execute with ability so delicate and so arduous a task. After passing several years at St. John's College, in Cambridge, in the pursuits of general science, he removed to Edinburgh to engage in the study of physic. But notwithstanding his acquisitions in the HEALING ART, to which he applied himself with great assiduity, he uniformly discovered a predilection for THEOLOGY. It became expedient, therefore, not to oppose the strong direction of his mind. He returned to Cambridge; and when he had taken the degree of LL. B. was admitted

admitted into holy orders. Being appointed to the chaplaincy of the British company of merchants, at St. Petersburgh, he removed thither; and executed the duties of that honourable and important station with exemplary fidelity, and with the general approbation of the factory. In this office he died, after a lingering and painful illness, on the 27th of May, 1798, in the thirty-second year of his age.

Note XXI. *Page* 127.

THE SALUTARY CONNECTIONS OF SICKNESS ARE NOT TO BE RASHLY DISSOLVED, BY REMOVING INTO AN HOSPITAL THOSE WHO MAY, WITH A LITTLE AID, ENJOY IN THEIR OWN HOMES, BENEFITS AND CONSOLATIONS, WHICH ELSEWHERE IT IS IN THE POWER OF NO ONE TO CONFER.

THE domestic benefits of sickness to the sufferer, and to his family, in fostering the tender attachments of affinity;—" the charities of father, son, and brother," are thus eloquently displayed by a late excellent divine.

" *Christian*, when, in the season *of sick-*" *ness*, you saw the solicitude of your friends: " the assiduity, perhaps, of a pious offspring " to

" to repay your care of them in doing for " you, what now you could do no longer " for yourself; when you observed their " anxiety, if any human care or intercession " could avail to snatch you from the impending " danger; when you saw them sacrificing ease, " and rest, and health, to administer to your " deliverance and comfort, holding nothing " dear to them, that if the will of God were " such, they might by any means restore you " and retain you; when you saw their zea- " lous care to do *all* to which their power ex- " tended; and their heartfelt anguish as to " that which their power could not reach; " when in their countenances you perceived " the alternate marks of hope and apprehen- " sion, of comfort and distress; while you saw " *all* this, while you experienced the benefits " and the consolations of their friendship, were " your hearts *so hard*, that such powerful at- " tachment, and such zealous service, could " draw forth from you no more than the *or-* " *dinary* current of affection? No, Christian, " surely that could not be. In such a situation, " the lightest expressions of sincere friendship, " come *full* upon the heart to a warmer wel- " come, and with more than ordinary weight. " When we are about to lose our blessings, " it

" it is then, perhaps, that we first see them in " their true importance. It is the same when " it seems to us that we are about to *leave* " them. The last conversation, the last kind " offices, the last mutual interchange of tender " words, and silent looks; that last scene, my " friends, will agitate the inmost heart, and " set open all the springs of sympathy and " benevolence. While that last scene is draw- " ing nigh, and as long, also, as the impression " of it remains in memory, every thing par- " takes of its tender influences. While the " heart is thus mollified, by the united power " of sharp affliction, and solemn expectation, " every kindness, every condolence, every good " wish, every even the lightest token of " benevolent attention, sinks deep into it. " The merit of our friends puts on an unusual " amiableness, and every thing we love is in- " expressibly endeared to us. Christians, ave " you ever felt these sentiments? If you have, " you cannot willingly abandon them; for as " surely as you have felt them, you approve " them. You would have loved yourselves " the better, if in all time past, *these* had on " all occasions been the abiding sentiments of " your hearts. The man who is as sensible as "he ought to be, and by a very little measure "of reflection might be, of what mighty use "may be made of such circumstances, and "their influences, to give pleasantness, ac- "ceptableness, and accuracy to his social du- "ties, not only within the more contracted "circle of his family and friends, but also in "the wider range of his benevolent affections, "will often be retracing these circumstances, "and their influences in his mind and heart, "that he may avail himself of them in the "services that he owes to the universal family "of God, and in the improvement of his own "soul, to a resemblance of the universal pa- "rent. In such cares, he will be the more "assiduous, if he will permit himself to think, "that the heart which has once been exposed "to such powerfully humanizing and attender- "ing influences, if it is not much the better, "must of necessity become much the worse for "them."*

* See Life of the Rev. Newcome Cappe, prefixed to his posthumous works, published by Mrs. C. Cappe, in 2 vol. 8vo. Page 48.

Note

Note XXII. *Page* 133.

DUTY OF HOSPITAL TRUSTEES IN ELECTING THE MEDICAL OFFICERS OF THE CHARITY.

On the 17th of March, 1798, the governors of the Salisbury Infirmary, published the following judicious advertisement, concerning the nomination of a physician to the charity:

"Whereas it is the common practice to " solicit votes on a vacancy of the offices of " physician, surgeon, apothecary, secretary, " &c. and as many and great inconveniencies " have frequently arisen from a too hasty com-" pliance with such solicitations, to the ex-" clusion of the most worthy candidates, and " the permanent detriment of the charity; and " as such inconsiderate promises may render " even the most judicious statutes and prudential " rules of any society ineffectual, it is hoped " that every governor of this charitable insti-" tution will, on all such occasions, keep him-" self entirely disengaged till the day of elec-" tion; and then, after a due examination into " the real merits of the candidates, give his " vote according to what he apprehends most " beneficial to that charity, of which he is the " guardian as well as the benefactor. The

 " reasonableness

" reasonableness of not promising votes will " be further evident, when it is considered " that such promises, previous to the day of " election, prevent perhaps him who is the " best qualified from appearing as a candidate, " well knowing it would be impossible for him " to succeed."

The following Memorial was presented, several years ago, to the trustees of the Manchester Infirmary; and the rule, recommended in it, has been ever since adopted.

" The medical committee, having been invited to lay before you their opinion concerning the qualifications requisite in your apothecary and house-surgeon, are naturally induced to extend their attention to the more important office, with which the physicians to these charities are invested. And they are persuaded you will feel, with them, an earnest solicitude that the vacancies, which now subsist, may hereafter be filled by men of approved respectability, and liberal education.

" By the established usage of the hospital, it is required, that every candidate for the office of physician, shall produce his DIPLOMA, for the inspection of the trustees; together with satisfactory attestations of his moral character, and professional endowments. In addition to these

these credentials, they conceive it to be highly expedient that he should deliver an extract, from the register of the university, of which he was a member; specifying the several branches of science which he has cultivated, and the period of his collegiate residence. Such a testimonial may always be claimed, and is generally in the possession of physicians who have been regularly educated: No candidate, therefore, who does not produce it, should be deemed eligible: For he thus tacitly acknowledges, that he has not enjoyed the requisite advantages of academical instruction; nor received his degree as the reward of legitimate examination, either during the course, or after the completion of his academical studies.

"No candidate having yet offered, nor any one being known to have the design of offering himself for either of the present medical vacancies in the hospital, the considerations they now take the liberty of suggesting to your serious attention, cannot even be suspected of personal reference, or invidious allusion. And they are conscious, on this occasion, of being actuated by a sincere desire to promote the best and most permanent interests of the institutions,

stitutions, with which, by your suffrages, they have the honour to be connected."

This memorial, under the form of a letter, having been presented to the trustees of the Manchester Infirmary, produced the two following resolutions:

1. The trustees are fully sensible of the importance of the considerations, which the physicians have stated to them, in the above letter; and feel an earnest solicitude that the present, and all future vacancies in the medical departments of the hospital, should be filled by men of liberal education, good moral character, and respectable professional endowments.

2. It was moved, seconded, and resolved unanimously, that it be recommended to every succeeding board, to send a copy of the preceding letter to every gentleman, who may offer himself a candidate for the office of physician to these charities.

www.ingramcontent.com/pod-product-compliance
Ingram Content Group UK Ltd.
Pitfield, Milton Keynes, MK11 3LW, UK
UKHW040657180125
453697UK00010B/240